Tools and Strategies for an Effective Hospitalist Program

Jeffrey R. Dichter, MD, FACP

Kenneth G. Simone, DO

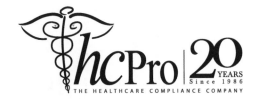

hcPro | 20 YEARS
Since 1986
THE HEALTHCARE COMPLIANCE COMPANY

Tools and Strategies for an Effective Hospitalist Program is published by HCPro, Inc.

Copyright 2006 HCPro, Inc.

All rights reserved. Printed in the United States of America.   5   4   3   2   1

ISBN 1-57839-766-9

No part of this publication may be reproduced, in any form or by any means, without prior written consent of HCPro, Inc. or the Copyright Clearance Center (978/750-8400). Please notify us immediately if you have received an unauthorized copy.

HCPro, Inc., provides information resources for the healthcare industry.

HCPro, Inc., is not affiliated in any way with the Joint Commission on Accreditation of Healthcare Organizations, which owns the JCAHO trademark.

Jeffrey R. Dichter, MD, FACP, Co-author
Kenneth G. Simone, DO, Co-author
Maureen Coler, Managing Editor
Matt Phillion, Associate Editor
Kathryn Levesque, Group Publisher
Jean St Pierre, Director of Operations
Jackie Diehl Singer, Graphic Artist
Laura Godinho, Cover Design
Paul Singer, Layout Artist

Advice given is general. Readers should consult professional counsel for specific legal, ethical, or clinical questions. Arrangements can be made for quantity discounts.

For more information, contact:

HCPro, Inc.
P.O. Box 1168
Marblehead, MA 01945
Telephone: 800/650-6787 or 781/639-1872
Fax: 781/639-2982
E-mail: *customerservice@hcpro.com*

Visit HCPro at its World Wide Web sites:
www.hcmarketplace.com and www.hcpro.com

3/2006
20747

CONTENTS

About the authors . . . . **viii**

Introduction . . . . **xii**

Chapter 1: Expectations for hospitalists **1**

Seek physicians' input 4

Let hospitalists know what they can expect in return 5

Keep job descriptions current 5

Tool: Figure 1.1: Description of hospitalist duties—Large academic medical

center with residents 7

Tool: Figure 1.2: Description of hospitalist duties—Small community

hospital without residents 12

Chapter 2: Staffing, scheduling, and planning **15**

Table 2.1: Sequence of practice development 18

Scheduling specifics 19

Coverage models 19

Scheduling mechanics 21

Tool: Figure 2.1: Four-hospitalist rotating call schedule—Variation 1 23

Tool: Figure 2.2: Four-hospitalist rotating call schedule—Variation 2 24

Tool: Figure 2.3: Four-hospitalist block schedule 25

Tool: Figure 2.4: Five-hospitalist block schedule—Variation 1 26

Tool: Figure 2.5: Five-hospitalist block schedule—Variation 2 27

Tool: Figure 2.6: Five-hospitalist seven days on/seven days off schedule 28

Tool: Figure 2.7: Six-hospitalist seven days on/seven days off schedule 30

Adjusting staffing levels using on-call back-up 31

Electronic solutions to scheduling 31

Tool: Figure 2.8: Protocol—Determining the need for on-call backup 32

Tool: Figure 2.9: Implementing an electronic, Internet-based solution to scheduling

multiple 24/7 shifts involving 30-plus hospitalists across two campuses 34

Chapter 3: Recruitment 35

Define your program 37

Characteristics of a hospitalist program practice 38

Candidates' observations about hospitalist programs 39

Include hospitalists' families in the recruitment process 40

The recruitment process and the recruitment checklist 41

Tool: Figure 3.1: The recruitment checklist 42

Chapter 4: Retention and orientation 49

Retention starts in the job interview 51

Question candidates with retention in mind 52

Survey new hospitalists 53

Employ a comprehensive orientation program 54

Tool: Figure 4.1: New physician retention interview 55

Tool: Figure 4.2: Orientation—Day #1 57

Tool: Figure 4.3: Orientation—Day #4 58

Notes 60

Chapter 5: The referring provider's perspective 61

Referring providers' expectations 63

Understanding the daily responsibilities of providers 64

What providers expect of hospitalists 64

What hospitalists can expect in return 65

Understanding the daily responsibilities of specialists 65

How specialists view hospitalists 66

Tool: Figure 5.1: The referring provider's 'wish list' for hospitalist services 67

Tool: Figure 5.2: The specialist's 'wish list' for hospitalist services 67

Chapter 6: Communication with healthcare practitioners 69

Communication modalities 72

The communication interface 75

Table Flow of information at patient discharge 81

Flow if information at discharge 81

Facilitating communication via electronic means 83

Communicating the admission protocol 83

Surveying referring providers 83

Surveying other providers 84

Tool: Figure 6.1: Establishing communication pathways via a Web-log 85

Tool: Figure 6.2: Communication between hospital and outpatient clinics in lieu

of an electronic medical records system 86

Tool: Figure 6.3: Admission protocol, including communication

expectations for hospitalists and referring providers .87

Tool: Figure 6.4: Referring physician satisfaction survey—Format 1 89

Tool: Figure 6.5: Referring physician satisfaction survey—Format 2 90

Tool: Figure 6.6: Referring physician satisfaction survey—Format 3 92

Tool: Figure 6.7: Nurse satisfaction survey—Format 1 94

Tool: Figure 6.8: Nurse satisfaction survey—Format 2 95

Chapter 7: Communication with patients 97

Measure patient satisfaction 100

Keep patient satisfaction out in the open 101

Marketing outreach for starting, expanding a hospitalist program 101

Tool: Figure 7.1: Patient satisfaction survey—Format 1 102

Tool: Figure 7.2: Patient satisfaction survey—Format 2 104

Tool: Figure 7.3: Draft communication plan for a hospitalist program launch 106

Tool: Figure 7.4: Letter to referring physicians announcing hospitalist

program launch 108

Tool: Figure 7.5: Draft communication plan for a hospitalist program expansion 110

Tool: Figure 7.6: Letter to referring physicians announcing hospitalist

program expansion 112

Develop a brochure to inform patients about the hospitalist service 113

Elements of a hospitalist brochure 113

Chapter 8: Hospitalist performance reviews 115

Changing culture 117

Roadblocks to evaluating performance 119

Clearly delineate expectations 119

Added benefits of conducting regular reviews 120

Tool: Figure 8.1: Departmental guidelines for evaluating
hospitalists' performance 121

Tool: Figure 8.2: Hospitalist performance evaluation—Format 1 122

Tool: Figure 8.3: Hospitalist performance evaluation—Format 2 127

Tool: Figure 8.4: Physician assistant performance evaluation 132

Chapter 9: Quality improvement and data collection 137

Quality measures 140

The balanced scorecard 141

Stretch targets 142

Relating compensation to quality of care 143

Generating a hospitalist report card 143

Tool: Figure 9.1: Hospitalist operational data and graphs 146

Frequency of reports 157

Tool: Figure 9.2: Operational data snapshot 158

Tool: Figure 9.3: Hospitalist report—Pneumonia core measures initiative 161

Tool: Figure 9.4: (Name of hospitalist service) quarterly report
(identify quarter) 164

Considerations when linking compensation to quality measures 170

References 171

Chapter 10: Preprinted orders 173

The development of preprinted orders 175

Guidelines for use 176

Solutions for tracking and organizing ordersets 177

Format and contents of ordersets 177

Tool: Figure 10.1: TNK (Tenecteplase—tPA) for myocardial infarction orders 179

Tool: Figure 10.2: Inpatient medical service physician's orders 180

Tool: Figure 10.3: Observation orders—Congestive heart failure 182

Tool: Figure 10.4: Observation orders—Chest pain 183

Tool: Figure 10.5: Observation orders—Asthma 184

Chapter 11: Coding and compliance for the inpatient physician 185

Current coding environment 187

Increased auditing activity 188

Challenges to determining the level of service 189

Table 11.1: Level 2 and level 3 admission comparison .192

Clinical examples 192

Table 11.2: Problem types associated with low-,moderate-, and
high-complexity medical decision-making 193

Table 11.3: Data to be ordered and/or reviewed 194

Table 11.4: Moderate-risk vs. high-risk examples 195

Table 11.5: Level 2 and level 3 subsequent hospital visit comparison 196

Differences between a level two and a level three subsequent hospital visit 196

Table 11.6: Differences between level three, four, and five consultations 197

Differences between level three, four, and five consultations 197

Table 11.7: Low-, medium-, and high-risk examples 198

Use of consultation codes 199

Critical care services 200

CPT changes for 2006 202

Online learning tools 203

CMS-sponsored E/M seminars 203

Physician Regulatory Issues Team (PRIT) 203

Helpful resources 203

About the Authors

Jeffrey R. Dichter, MD, FACP

Jeffrey R. Dichter, MD, FACP, a practicing hospitalist and internist, is a partner of Medical Consultants, PC, a large multi-specialty group in Muncie, IN. Dichter is a previous president of the Society of Hospital Medicine and the original director and founder of the hospital medicine program at Ball Memorial Hospital, also in Muncie. He earned his undergraduate degree from the University of California, Berkeley, and graduated from the medical school at the University of Southern California, Los Angeles. Dichter is board certified in both internal medicine and critical care medicine. His internal medicine training was completed at Los Angeles County General Hospital and his critical care fellowship at the National Institutes of Health in Bethesda, MD. Effective July 2006, he will be the director of the Critical Care Service at Presbyterian Hospital in Albuquerque, NM.

Kenneth G. Simone, DO

Kenneth G. Simone, DO, is a board-certified family physician in private family practice in Brewer, ME, and a founding member and vice president of the largest primary care group practice in greater Bangor. He is founder and president of Hospitalist and Practice Solutions, which specializes in hospitalist program development. Simone is the past president of the medical staff at St. Joseph Hospital in Bangor. He founded the oldest hospitalist program in Maine and served as its administrative director for 10 years. He sits on the editorial advisory board for two national hospitalist publications, and presently serves on the boards of the University of New England and the Medical Network of Maine. He earned his undergraduate degree from Boston College and graduated from New England College of Osteopathic Medicine.

Contact the authors

Jeffrey R. Dichter, MD, FACP

Partner, Medical Consultants, PC

Founder, Hospital Medicine Program

Ball Memorial Hospital

Previous President, Society of Hospital Medicine (2003–2004)

2525 University Avenue, Suite 300

Muncie, IN 47303

jrdichter@iquest.net

Kenneth G. Simone, DO

Founder and President, Hospitalist and Practice Solutions

Past President of the Medical Staff, St. Joseph Hospital

Founder, Northeast Inpatient Medical Services

42 Silver Ridge

Veazie, ME 04401

ksimone@sunburypc.com

Contact the contributing authors

Alpesh N. Amin, MD, MBA, FACP

Executive Director, Hospitalist Program

Vice Chair for Clinical Affairs & Quality, Dept. of Medicine

Associate Program Director, Internal Medicine Residents

University of California, Irvine

101 The City Drive South, Bldg. 58

Room 110, ZC-4076H

Orange CA 92868

anamin@uci.edu

Diane Craig, MD, FACP

Assistant Physician-in-Chief

The Permanente Medical Group

710 Lawrence Expressway

Santa Clara, CA 95051

diane.craig@kp.org

Sylvia C. W. McKean, MD, FACP

Medical Director

Brigham and Women's Hospital/Faulkner Hospitalist Service

PBB-B, Suite 428, Room 429

15 Francis St.

Boston, MA 02115

smckean@partners.org

Charleen A. Porter, BS, MA, CPC

Billing & Coding Consultant

VEI Community Health Network

7240 Shadeland Station, Suite 300

Indianapolis, IN 46256

caporter@insightbb.com

Richard E. Rohr, MD, FACP

Director of Hospitalists

Milford Hospital

Department of Internal Medicine

300 Seaside Ave.

Milford, CT 06460

richard.rohr@milfordhospital.org

Greg Susla, PharmD, FCCM

Pharmacy Manager

VHA, Inc.

5301 Hines Road

Frederick, MD 21704

gsusla@vha.com

Contact the tools contributors

Brian J. Bossard, MD

Director, Inpatient Physician Associates

2300 S. 16th Street

Lincoln, NE 68502

brian.bossard@bryanlgh.org

Jenifir Bruno, MD

FirstHealth Moore Regional Hospital

155 Memorial Drive

Pinehurst, NC 28374

jbruno@firsthealth.org

Mary Dallas, MD

Medical Information Officer

Presbyterian Health System

P.O. Box 26666

Albuquerque, NM 87125

mdallas@phs.org

Revathi A-Davidson, MPH

Program Administrator for the Hospitalist Group

Presbyterian Health System

P.O. Box 26666

Albuquerque, NM 87125

rdavidso@phs.org

Mary Jo Gorman, MD, MBA

Chief Medical Officer, IPC—The Hospitalist Company

President-elect, Society of Hospital Medicine

4605 Lankershim Blvd., Suite 617

North Hollywood, CA 91602

mjgorman@ipcm.com

INTRODUCTION

Over the past 15 years, the field of hospital medicine has grown dramatically. The number of hospitalists and programs recruiting these professionals has grown exponentially. In fact, few if any programs are *not* actively recruiting new hospitalists. Although the specialty is growing rapidly, however, the demand for quality hospitalists is surpassing the supply. As a result, hospitalist program directors are faced with the task of providing high-quality services while managing an impossible workload.

As hospital medicine programs contend with the "consequences" of their success, the expectations and roles of hospitalists increase and expand. The healthcare industry has tasked hospitalists with being leaders in the delivery of safe, quality, efficient, and cost-effective hospital medical care and is grading them based on performance and patient satisfaction measures. Under the pressures of these added expectations, hospitalists' workloads are daunting, if not completely overwhelming.

Therefore, to accomplish non-clinical-care missions, hospitalist programs require administrative support. The administrative support available to a program correlates with its ability to create processes that provide structure and feedback regarding the program's overall performance. Some of these processes include

1. developing protocols for hospitalists' communication with referring physicians, other healthcare professionals, patients, families, and others

2. developing new call schedules as programs add new hospitalists

3. collecting, tracking, and monitoring data regarding quality measures, efficiency measures, and patient satisfaction rates, among other data

4. refining a successful recruitment process and ensuring that there are adequate personnel resources to support it

5. developing a comprehensive orientation process for new hospitalists

 © 2006 HCPRO, INC. **TOOLS AND STRATEGIES FOR AN EFFECTIVE HOSPITALIST PROGRAM**

These processes, or "tools," are quickly becoming necessary for most hospitalist programs. In our experience, maintaining the necessary administrative support to develop crucial processes allows programs to develop tools that optimize successful outcomes while minimizing wasted time and energy. Furthermore, we believe that programs are more effective and efficient when they have access to more well-developed tools to use. However, creating these tools requires a great deal of work, and few programs have the resources to develop them beyond a basic form.

In undertaking this project, it was our goal to reach out to programs nationwide that were willing to share their tools, gather the ones that they felt were essential to their programs' success, and share as many as possible with our readers. The result is a hands-on tools book that we hope provides you with a solid foundation on which to build or reformulate a hospitalist program dedicated to quality care and patient satisfaction.

This collection of tools is provided in standard published format as well as on the accompanying CD-ROM so that you may download, print, modify, and distribute them as needed. The tools are meant to serve as a guide and can be customized to fit any hospitalist program.

We are grateful to the many programs that shared their tools for this publication. This book would not have been possible without their talents in developing these outstanding tools and their willingness to share them with others. The more successful individual hospitalist programs are, the more successful our entire specialty of hospital medicine will become—and, ultimately, our patients are the greatest benefactors of our successes.

—Jeffrey R. Dichter, MD, FACP
—Kenneth G. Simone, DO

Expectations for hospitalists

1

Expectations for hospitalists

Alpesh N. Amin, MD, MBA, FACP

Richard E. Rohr, MD, FACP

Hospital administrations are demanding ever-higher levels of performance by physicians while placing them under greater scrutiny. Physicians' roles as clinicians have never before been so regulated, monitored, and analyzed.

A host of factors may be contributing to this trend, including the following:

- The healthcare industry's focus on improving individual physician performance
- The general public's and the government's increasing interest in high-quality patient care
- The increasing involvement of physicians on various quality and safety committees and in the peer-review process

The increasing scrutiny is especially true for hospitalists who—in their roles as the "hubs" of inpatient clinical care—find their job expectations expanding constantly to include tasks relevant to the business side of medicine (e.g., decreasing the length of hospital stays, becoming documentation experts to maximize hospital reimbursement, etc.).

Hospitalists are generally committed to doing a good job at everything they do. That's part of what drew them to medicine in the first place. Once hospitalists know what is expected of them, they provide it with 110% effort—provided that they are 100% aware of all that is expected of them.

To expect physicians to fulfill their responsibilities, but not to orient them to these duties, sets them up to fail. If you want to help your hospitalists perform successfully in their clinical and other staff leadership roles, develop a written job description for each role (e.g., clinical, medical staff leadership) they will fulfill. This is a basic function of establishing and communicating clear expectations.

The following are examples of the basic elements in a comprehensive job description for hospitalists:

- The identity of the individual (and perhaps department) to whom the hospitalist is accountable

- A clear listing of the hospitalist's responsibilities as a hospitalist

- A definition of the expectations of the hospitalist for each responsibility

- An explanation of the review process and a timeline for evaluating the hospitalist's performance

- A set of clear expectations about long-term goals and quality standards

Remember, the expectations listed on the hospitalist's job description can be used to measure performance at evaluation time provided that they are current, objective, and measurable.

Seek physicians' input

Secure the medical staff's and the institution's support when determining the hospitalist's duties and responsibilities, both in terms of the clinical aspects of the job and with regard to behavioral and cultural expectations. The best way to cultivate hospitalist buy-in is to encourage and solicit physicians' input in creating and updating the job description and expectations.

If your facility does not yet have a written job description defining hospitalists' expectations, the following steps will guide you in creating one.

1. Educate current hospitalists and other appropriate medical staff members about the need for a written job description or policy.

2. Appoint a task force to draft an initial set of hospitalist performance expectations. In essence, this task asks hospitalists to personally define what it means to be a "good" physician.

3. When it is still in draft form, make the job description or policy an explicit agenda item for discussion in a medical staff meeting (for each relevant department). Regardless of the approach your department or staff members take, hospitalists' expectations must be shared with all medical staff members. Seek out opportunities to discuss the draft with hospitalists in the hallways, in the operating room lounge, and even in social settings.

4. Implement the expectations, ensuring that all hospitalists currently on staff have a copy and that incoming hospitalists receive a copy with their orientation materials.

Let hospitalists know what they can expect in return

Remember that defining clear expectations is a two-way street. Your organization must let hospitalists know what they can expect in return for their good work. For example, perhaps your facility is willing to provide additional support staff members (e.g., case managers, physician assistants) when the hospitalists' workload reaches a certain threshold. Or, perhaps your program will accommodate physicians by offering them more flexible schedules when possible.

Keep job descriptions current

Today's rapidly changing healthcare environment also mandates that job descriptions and on-the-job expectations are kept current. This is especially true for hospitalists, whose roles continue to evolve. For example, in many institutions, it is becoming more common for hospitalists to take a role in comanaging pre-operative and post-operative patients. There is also a growing expectation that hospitalists will make second daily visits to patients under their care.

Other expectations of hospitalists that your organization may consider include responsibility for

• staffing rapid response and code teams

- serving on or chairing various hospital committees
- providing training and education to key hospital personal (e.g., nurses, technicians, etc.)
- covering patients at more than one hospital or site

In addition, hospitalists at your facility might be involved in oversight of utilization data, improving program efficiency (e.g., length of stay, patient flow, readmission rates), developing clinical protocols, or teaching medical students and residents.

Because job descriptions evolve over time, ensure that even those hospitalists who are veterans of the program are provided with an up-to-date, detailed job description or job expectations policy.

The following figures are sample job descriptions. **Figure 1.1** is an example of a comprehensive job description for a hospitalist in an inpatient medicine program at a large, academic medical center where hospitalists may have responsibilities for teaching medical residents. **Figure 1.2** is a description of hospitalists' duties at a small community hospital without residents.

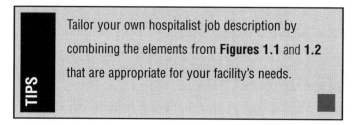

TIPS

Tailor your own hospitalist job description by combining the elements from **Figures 1.1** and **1.2** that are appropriate for your facility's needs.

Description of hospitalist duties: Large academic medical center with residents

A. *(Name of hospitalist service)* **hospitalist general job description**

- Perform rounds Monday through Friday, taking full ownership of the general internal medicine inpatient service during weekday business hours.

- Perform internal medicine consultations.

- Participate (occasionally) in the ambulatory clinic, which may include private practice, preoperative clinic, same day, urgent care, post-hospital follow-up, procedure, and/or clinic attending responsibility.

- Attend regular meetings with the executive director of the hospitalist program.

- Attend/participate in the monthly hospitalist program faculty meeting.

- Attend/participate in the department of medicine faculty meetings.

- Attend/participate in the division of general internal medicine meetings.

- Become actively involved in various administrative committees and projects as determined by the executive director of the hospitalist program.

- Follow the hospitalist program policies on patient care, availability, medical education/teaching, and academics.

- Become an integral part of the hospitalist team and be willing to provide backup as needed.

- Participate in evening and weekend call as scheduled by the hospitalist program.

B. *(Name of hospitalist service)* **hospitalist inpatient responsibilities**

As a *(name of hospitalist service)* hospitalist, you will provide inpatient services at *(name of hospital)*. You will also provide on-call weekend coverage, which will be rotated among the participating hospitalists. On-call coverage may include performing rounds on the weekend, facilitating transfers, and taking and documenting telephone calls from patients and physicians. Along with other members of the hospitalist faculty, you will be responsible for carrying the hospitalist beeper.

Figure 1.1 Description of hospitalist duties: Large academic medical center with residents (cont.)

The duties and responsibilities for ward attending and consult services include the following:

- Establishing and maintaining primary attending responsibility for inpatient general internal medicine service.

- Providing leadership and education to the entire care team.

- Working with case managers to ensure appropriate length of stay, efficient use of resources, and appropriate follow-up care.

- Providing direct patient care to general internal medicine patients.

- Meeting with families and maintaining a presence on the ward.

- Directly supervising residents and medical students on the general internal medicine services.

- Conducting teaching rounds for fellows, residents, and medical students.

- Reviewing (daily or more frequently) all of the patients on your service with fellows, house staff, and students, as needed.

- Serving as role model for your students, house staff, and fellows.

- Serving as a liaison to referring physicians—both *(name of hospital)* and non-*(name of hospital)* to facilitate the growth of the inpatient service.

- Understanding, implementing, and teaching quality and optimum utilization of services.

- Developing appropriate inpatient clinical pathways.

- Dictating all histories/physicals, progress notes, procedure notes, consult notes, consult follow-ups, and discharge notes.

- Leading and attending daily review conferences on your patients as appropriate.

- Supervising all planned discharges for appropriateness and timeliness.

Description of hospitalist duties: Large academic medical center with residents (cont.)

- Working daily with case managers to provide appropriate and timely use of resources (ensuring appropriate and timely use of diagnostic and ancillary services).

- Ensuring proper communication to the primary care physician and specialists.

C. *(Name of hospitalist service)* **hospitalist outpatient responsibilities**

1. Resident and fellow supervision duties

You will be responsible for the supervision of any students, residents, and fellows who may rotate through the hospitalist clinics. A session includes all the time required to complete patient care coordination and charting. The duties and responsibilities in the hospitalist clinic are as follows:

- Supervise residents.

- See all patients briefly to ensure appropriateness of care and to demonstrate/establish the role of attending physicians to patients.

- See all scheduled patients if there are no residents or fellows.

- Ensure that students, residents, and fellows practice efficiently.

- Serve as a role model and mentor for assigned students, residents, and fellows.

- Participate in any appropriate utilization protocols.

- Arrive on time at the start of each scheduled attending session.

- Do not leave until all patients under your supervision have been discharged.

- Document all visits in the patient's medical record.

- Co-sign the billing sheet and ensure that procedure and diagnosis codes are entered correctly.

- Ensure that the resident and fellow physicians finish prescribing all medication refills, chart checks, forms, etc., before they leave.

Figure 1.1 Description of hospitalist duties: Large academic medical center with residents (cont.)

• Submit requests for time off in writing to the hospitalist program executive director.

2. Direct patient care

• Arrive on time

• Do not leave when you still have patients in the room.

• Sign all lab and radiology reports daily for your patients and patients of providers who are out of the office.

• Review (daily) all requests for prescriptions.

• Complete normal lab letter for all labs.

• Answer pages.

• Cooperate in covering for absent colleagues (labs, prescriptions, phone calls, etc.).

• Sign the billing sheet, and ensure that procedure and diagnosis codes are correctly entered.

• Submit requests for time off in writing to the hospitalist program executive director.

   D. *(Name of hospitalist service)* **hospitalist administrative time**

You will be expected to follow general hospitalist program policies regarding your administrative duties as determined in conjunction with the hospitalist program executive director. Appropriate use of any administrative time can be used for the following types of activities:

• Development, implementation, and monitoring of clinical pathways and quality improvement projects

• Completion of medical records, etc.

• Hospitalist program administrative projects

• Peer review, utilization, and quality improvement activities as assigned

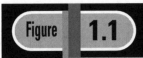

Figure 1.1 Description of hospitalist duties: Large academic medical center with residents (cont.)

- Resident and medical student educational activities

- Curriculum development and lecture preparation

- Continuing medical education self-study

- Practice site administrative activities as assigned

- Required meetings

- Hospitalist research and academic projects

Physicians' administrative activities may be assigned at the discretion of the hospitalist program and hospitalist program executive director. Administrative time is not to be taken as time off.

While performing administrative activities, hospitalist faculty must be available by pager and be available for backup as needed.

Source: **Alpesh N. Amin, MD, MBA, FACP,** *executive director of the hospitalist program, vice chair for clinical affairs and quality, and associate program director of internal medicine residents, Department of Medicine at the University of California, Irvine, CA.*

Figure 1.2 — Description of hospitalist duties: Small community hospital without residents

Expectations for *(name of hospital/hospitalist service)* **hospitalists:**

To whom the expectations apply: This set of expectations is designed for hospitalists in a small community hospital without residents, where the hospitalists cover the intensive care unit and other areas of the hospital. Some of the expectations may need to be modified for other hospitals. By articulating the level of performance expected in each dimension, the job description becomes a tool for managing physician performance.

Prospective and new hires: Candidates for employment should be evaluated on their ability to meet the expectations. All new hires should be given the expectations on their first day of work. Subsequent evaluations should be based on how well the individual meets expectations. This method has proven successful in reducing the amount of time spent on managing poor performance.

Additional (quantitative) considerations: Specific measurements should be developed for all quantitative dimensions of performance (e.g., percentage of patients receiving pneumonia vaccine, patient satisfaction scores, number of committee meetings attended).

Subjective measures: The quality of relations with patients, physicians, and other health professionals requires a subjective assessment by the manager. Relationships with others can be judged in part by considering complaints received, but this will not capture the positive aspects of those relationships, and some additional probing by the manager is required for a balanced assessment.

Technical quality:

- Achieve and maintain certification by the American Board of Internal Medicine.

- Maintain membership on the hospital medical staff.

- Complete 50 hours of accredited continuing medical education annually in topics related to inpatient medicine.

- Achieve and maintain certification by the American Heart Association in advanced cardiac life support.

12 ■ © 2006 HCPRO, INC. TOOLS AND STRATEGIES FOR AN EFFECTIVE HOSPITALIST PROGRAM

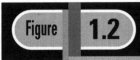

Figure 1.2 — Description of hospitalist duties: Small community hospital without residents (cont.)

Life support:

- Achieve and maintain proficiency in endotracheal intubation.

Service quality:

- Provide prompt responses to calls from nursing units and the emergency department.

- Maintain friendly relations with patients and families and avoid confrontations.

Productivity:

- Complete evaluations of all admissions and other patients prior to the completion of your shift.

- Assess utilization of intensive care and telemetry beds during your shift, and avoid holding patients in the emergency department.

Resource utilization:

- Comply with clinical guidelines adopted by the hospital relating to disease management, medications, and testing.

Co-worker relations:

- Develop positive relations with community physicians, emergency physicians, nurses, case managers, and other staff.

- Resolve conflicts with physicians and co-workers in a quiet and professional manner.

- Respond positively to suggestions from physician and non-physician co-workers.

Organizational commitment:

- Participate in quality improvement activities and hospital committees.

Source: Richard E. Rohr, MD, FACP, director of the hospitalist service at Milford (CT) Hospital.

Staffing, scheduling, and planning

2

Staffing, scheduling, and planning

Kenneth G. Simone, DO

Developing a hospitalist schedule is a unique process for each program. It is based on the organization's objectives and mission, financial resources, and staffing availability. Successful programs each typically develop a strategic plan and timeline to allow for controlled growth and concomitant adjustments in the practice structure.

A hospitalist program should first establish its objectives and mission by evaluating

- community needs
- the organization's overall mission
- medical staff resources and desires
- healthcare competition
- the customer base

It also should consider stabilizing the primary care and specialty referral network. Once these objectives and the mission are defined, the program should delineate the scope of deliverable services. The hospitalist structure and schedule can then be altered to accommodate the program at each stage of implementation. For example, a hospitalist program may first offer daytime coverage (7 a.m. to 5 p.m.) for community primary care physicians (PCP) and then slowly progress to a 24/7 model that enables the service to accept all referrals. Be aware that coverage changes may require alterations in the staffing model and structure.

When evaluating the merits of various practice models (e.g., seven days on and seven days off, 36-hour shifts, block scheduling, or some other arrangement), consider continuity of care, anticipated volume/census, and the added-value services (e.g., staffing rapid response teams, training/educating key hospital personnel) your hospitalist program will offer to the institution. The program should advocate providers' participation in various strategic hospital committees and initiatives. Considerations also include time allotted for a hospitalist's vacation, continuing medical education (CME), sick time, and maternity leave. A premium should be placed on the model that will maximize recruitment and retention at your facility.

Practice stability is essential to any successful hospitalist program. The staffing and scheduling plan should consider the hospitalist service's and the organization's short- and long-term strategic goals, marketing plan, and program structure. **Table 2.1** below is a flow chart demonstrating the sequence of hospitalist practice development and the relationship between the key components that ensure practice stability.

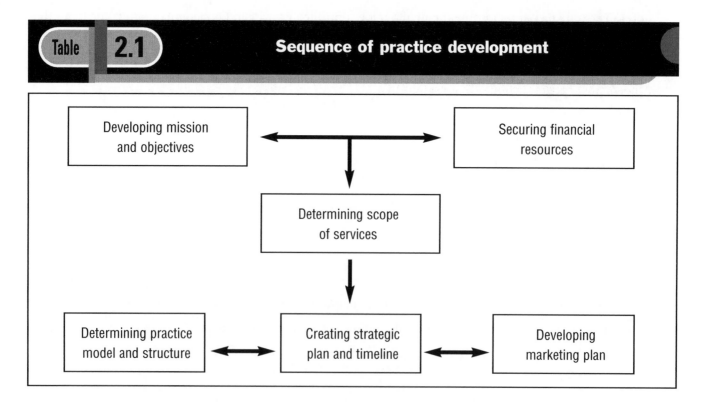

| Table **2.1** | **Sequence of practice development** |

Developing mission and objectives ←→ Securing financial resources

Determining scope of services

Determining practice model and structure ←→ Creating strategic plan and timeline ←→ Developing marketing plan

Staffing, scheduling, and planning

2

The schedule is important to the lifestyle concerns of the providers and may be vital to preventing burnout. The marketing plan should complement the anticipated growth and staffing needs. The expansion of the practice must conform to an increase in the referral and patient base to ensure practice sustainability for the long term.

Scheduling specifics

When deciding on a provider schedule, examine many options. Factors driving the decision include the depth of coverage the program will provide, the desired practice model, and staff size.

Staff size is influenced by the assumptions made at the onset of the program. You can develop a schedule based on one of several factors, including staffing based on census, number of admissions and consultations per year, encounters per year, and clinical hours worked per provider per year. Again, do not forget to factor in the added-value services the practice will deliver.

Coverage models

The following is a review of various coverage and practice models. You can choose from many variations to customize your schedule.

Daytime coverage

Daytime coverage is typically defined as 7 a.m. to 5 p.m. coverage. The hospitalist conducts daily rounds on all patients on the practice service and conducts all admissions that occur during these hours. Referring physicians that use the hospitalist service provide the night call. Another option is to have the hospitalist participate in the nighttime call on a regular rotating basis with the same frequency as the outpatient physicians. This requires the least amount of staffing (i.e., dedicated hospitalists), is cost effective, and maintains continuity of care. However, it is often the least desirable model for referring providers because they are responsible for participating in night call.

24/7 coverage

This model is a full-time hospitalist program that does not require full-time in-hospital presence. The practice is responsible for covering itself 24 hours per day/365 days a year. Most mature hospitalist programs provide this scope of coverage.

24/7 in-house coverage

This model is a full-time hospitalist program that requires in-house hospitalist presence 24 hours per day/365 days a year. Staffing requirements are typically greater for this type of coverage. Hospitalists who are part of these programs usually become an integral part of rapid response and code teams due to their around-the-clock hospital presence.

'Traditional' call

This coverage arrangement requires all members of the practice to cover night call on a regular rotating basis. Thus, the hospitalist frequently works a 36-hour shift. Some practices enable the hospitalist to go home early after making rounds the morning following call. This model is cost effective, maintains continuity of care, facilitates strong communication lines, and enables flexibility in scheduling. The disadvantage is that night call and weekends can be overwhelmingly busy. Quality-of-life concerns are not truly addressed with traditional call, making it one of the least attractive models for hospitalists. Further, this schedule may lead to hospitalist burnout and increased staff turnover.

Block scheduling

According to this scheduling arrangement, multiple providers work days, one or two providers work nights, and some combination of providers works during the weekend. This schedule allows for 12- to 14-hour shifts and, typically (e.g., in a six-person practice or larger), no physician is required to take "call" (i.e., work 24 or 36 hours). The hospitalists' schedules are "blocked" so that each works for four to 14 consecutive days, followed by a number of days off. The schedule typically rotates so each hospitalist covers days, nights, and weekends throughout the year. The blocks usually rotate every two to six weeks. The advantages of this model include continuity of care, lack of call (hospitalists do not carry their beepers when their shift is completed), and increased availability, which fosters communication and efficient case management. The disadvantages include a decrease in scheduling flexibility, decreased cost effectiveness, and the potential for provider burnout and turnover.

Shift work

Shift work is often confused with block scheduling, but it is a distinct model in which providers are scheduled to work a day, evening, or night shift. The shifts may vary from day to day, and a hospitalist's work schedule may be fragmented (e.g., no consecutive shifts). A similar model works well in the emergency department but has many weaknesses when applied to hospitalist programs. Advantages of this schedule include the elimination of a need for call, flexibility in scheduling, and predictability for hospitalists. The primary disadvantages include discontinuity of care, loss of teamwork and practice camaraderie, potential disruption in communication, and cost inefficiency.

Seven days on/seven days off

With this schedule, hospitalists are divided into two or three teams depending on practice size. They are scheduled to work for seven consecutive days followed by seven consecutive days off. Typically, the workweek concludes with a 24-hour shift. The team rotation is staggered so that all hospitalists do not change at one time. An individual is assigned to night call. All providers rotate into the night call slot throughout the year. This model appears to provide continuity, and many physicians are attracted to it for lifestyle purposes. They work 26 weeks each year and have 26 weeks off. Although it may be slightly less cost effective (because at any given time only half the providers are working), this structure can save money because it can increase recruitment, retention, and stability of physicians. The disadvantages of this model are that the physicians may not be available to provide the added-value services on their weeks off. Additionally, scheduling flexibility and communication decline.

Scheduling mechanics

Once you have made a decision about the number of hospitalists a program will employ (full time and part time), select a practice model and build a schedule. During this process, consider the following:

- Practice mission and objectives
- Financial resources
- Community needs
- Medical staff resources and desires
- Referral and customer base
- Projected patient census
- Stability of primary care physician and specialist networks
- Maintenance of continuity of care
- Communication (among hospitalists and to PCPs)
- Schedule flexibility
- Recruitment and retention
- Added-value services

Several of these items—mission, objectives, and community needs—are fixed following the planning process, while others—census, staffing, and financial resources—are dynamic and variable.

This is an important concept to remember because it can alter the practice model and schedule in the future. Successful hospitalist programs have the vision and flexibility to be proactive and make necessary adjustments as these variables and resources change over time.

The schedule variations we provide in **Figures 2.1–2.7** assume a one-hospital system with a stable census and fixed financial resources. In addition, we assume that no monies will be allocated in the budget for hiring locum tenens (i.e., temporary) physicians or part-time employees—meaning that there is no flexibility in staffing for vacations, sick time, continuing medical education (CME), etc. Thus, the schedule must work based on its own merits.

The hospitalists are given four weeks vacation (including sick time) and one week CME, and the program factors in time for the added-value benefits it provides to the hospital. **Figures 2.1–2.7** are variations of a four, five, or six full-time provider hospitalist practice. Adding a seventh full-time hospitalist to these schedules requires minimal change.

Four-hospitalist rotating call schedule—Variation 1

Figure 2.1 demonstrates an example of a four-hospitalist rotating call schedule.

Four-hospitalist rotating call schedule—Variation 2

Figure 2.2 demonstrates a second variation of a four-hospitalist rotating call schedule.

Four-hospitalist block schedule

Figure 2.3 demonstrates a four-hospitalist block schedule.

Five-hospitalist block schedule—Variation 1

Figure 2.4 demonstrates a block schedule using five hospitalists.

Five-hospitalist block schedule—Variation 2

Figure 2.5 demonstrates a second variation of a block schedule using five hospitalists.

Five-hospitalist seven days on/seven days off schedule

Figure 2.6 shows a schedule in which, on average, a hospitalist works seven consecutive days, ending each workweek with a 24-hour shift.

Six-hospitalist seven days on/seven days off schedule

Figure 2.7 is a schedule using six hospitalists in a seven-days-on and seven-days-off model.

Four-hospitalist rotating call schedule—Variation 1

Week 1	Mon.	Tues.	Wed.	Thurs.	Fri.	Sat.	Sun.
Day	A, B, C	A, B, C	A, B, C	A, B, C	A, B, C	A, B	A, B
Night	B	C	A	B	C	B	A
Week 2	B, C, D	B, C, D	B, C, D	B, C, D	B, C, D	C, D	C, D
Day	D	B	C	D	B	D	C
Night							
Week 3	A, B, D	A, B, D	A, B, D	A, B, D	A, B, D	A, B	A, B
Day	A	D	B	A	D	A	B
Night							
Week 4	A, C, D	A, C, D	A, C, D	A, C, D	A, C, D	C, D	C, D
Day	C	A	D	C	A	C	D
Night							

Figure 2.1 demonstrates one option for a four-hospitalist rotating call schedule. In this scheme, only three providers work each week. This schedule enables each hospitalist to have one week "off " per four-week month.

The hospitalists rotate call every third night (when they are not on their weeks off), as well as every other weekend. This schedule provides some flexibility (because the fourth physician is not scheduled) and enables the practice to provide added-value benefits to the hospital. It also may enable the hospitalists to pursue other areas of interest, such as research or work at subspecialty clinics.

Continuity appears to be maintained throughout the weekends. The disadvantage of this model is that the hospitalists typically work 36-hour shifts multiple times in a week.

*Source: **Kenneth G. Simone, DO,** founder and president, Hospitalist and Practice Solutions, Veazie, ME.*

Figure **2.2**   **Four-hospitalist rotating call schedule—Variation 2**

Week 1	Mon.	Tues.	Wed.	Thurs.	Fri.	Sat.	Sun.
Day	A, B, C	A, B, D	B, C, D	A, C, D	A, B, C	A, B	A, B
Night	C	A	B	D	C	A	B
Week 2							
Day	A, C, D	B, C, D	A, B, C	A, B, D	A, B,C	C, D	C, D
Night	A	D	C	B	A	D	C
Week 3							
Day	A, B, D	A, B, C	A, C, D	B, C, D	A, B, D	A, B	A, B
Night	D	B	A	C	D	B	A
Week 4							
Day	B, C, D	A, C, D	A, B, D	A, B, C	B, C, D	C, D	C, D
Night	B	C	D	A	B	C	D

Figure 2.2 demonstrates a second variation of a four-hospitalist rotating call schedule. In this model, all four hospitalists work each week. This schedule decreases the flexibility of the staff, but the physicians are typically on call every fourth night (rather than every third night).

This variation eliminates the 36-hour shift except for weekend call. Following weekday call, the hospitalist performs rounds on his or her patients and checks out to the hospitalist who is on call that evening.

Continuity appears to be maintained throughout the weekends. The disadvantage is that there is no built-in mechanism to handle unforeseen problems with a hospitalist (e.g., a hospitalist is sick or otherwise unable to report to work). Additionally, it may be difficult to provide added-value services (e.g., staffing rapid response teams) with such a tight schedule.

*Source: **Kenneth G. Simone, DO,** founder and president, Hospitalist and Practice Solutions, Veazie, ME.*

Figure 2.3 — Four-hospitalist block schedule

Week 1	Mon.	Tues.	Wed.	Thurs.	Fri.	Sat.	Sun.
Day	A, B, C	A, B, C	A, B, C	A, B, C	A, B, C	A, B	A, B
Night	D	D	D	D	D	A	B
Week 2							
Day	B, C, D	B, C, D	B, C, D	B, C, D	B, C, D	C, D	C, D
Night	A	A	A	A	A	C	D
Week 3							
Day	A, B, D	A, B, D	A, B, D	A, B, D	A, B, D	A, B	A, B
Night	C	C	C	C	C	B	A
Week 4							
Day	A, C, D	A, C, D	A, C, D	A, C, D	A, C, D	C, D	C, D
Night	B	B	B	B	B	D	C

Figure 2.3 demonstrates a four-hospitalist block schedule that maintains continuity but requires hospitalists to perform a 36-hour shift on weekends. This may negate the positives of a block schedule model that is typically designed to eliminate the rugged 36-hour shifts. The providers are on every other weekend.

The positive aspect of this schedule is that the daytime hospitalists have no call on weekdays. Note that the flexibility of a block schedule is compromised with only four physicians.

Source: **Kenneth G. Simone, DO,** *founder and president, Hospitalist and Practice Solutions, Veazie, ME.*

| Figure | 2.4 | Five-hospitalist block schedule—Variation 1 |

Week 1	Mon.	Tues.	Wed.	Thurs.	Fri.	Sat.	Sun.
Day	A, B, C	A, B, C	A, B, C	A, B, C	A, B, C	A, B	A, B
Night	D	D	D	D	D	A	B
Week 2							
Day	A, C, E	A, C, E	A, C, E	A, C, E	A, C, E	C, E	C, E
Night	B	B	B	B	B	E	C
Week 3							
Day	A, D, E	A, D, E	A, D, E	A, D, E	A, D, E	A, D	A, D
Night	C	C	C	C	C	D	A
Week 4							
Day	B, D, E	B, D, E	B, D, E	B, D, E	B, D, E	B, E	B, E
Night	A	A	A	A	A	B	E
Week 5							
Day	B, C, D	B, C, D	B, C, D	B, C, D	B, C, D	C, D	C, D
Night	E	E	E	E	E	C	D

Figure 2.4 demonstrates one variation of a block schedule using five hospitalists. In this model, only four of the five hospitalists work each week. All of the hospitalists work in 12-day blocks.

This schedule maintains continuity of care and provides flexibility. Hospitalists have a week off after their week of nights. Each physician works two nonconsecutive weekends in every five, as well as only one 36-hour shift and one 24-hour shift every five weeks. The other shifts are 12 hours in duration.

This schedule enables the hospitalist program to provide the hospital with added-value services (e.g., staffing rapid response or code teams, providing training and education to key hospital personnel).

*Source: **Kenneth G. Simone, DO,** founder and president, Hospitalist and Practice Solutions, Veazie, ME.*

| Figure | 2.5 | Five-hospitalist block schedule—Variation 2 |

Week 1	Mon.	Tues.	Wed.	Thurs.	Fri.	Sat.	Sun.
Day	A, B, E	A, B, E	A, B, E	A, B, E	A, B, C	A, C	A, C
Night	D	D	D	D	D	E	E
Week 2							
Day	A, B, C	A, B, C	A, B, C	A, B, C	B, C, D	B, D	B, D
Night	E	E	E	E	E	A	A
Week 3							
Day	B, C, D	B, C, D	B, C, D	B, C, D	C, D, E	C, E	C, E
Night	A	A	A	A	A	B	B
Week 4							
Day	C, D, E	C, D, E	C, D, E	C, D, E	A, D, E	A, D	A, D
Night	B	B	B	B	B	C	C
Week 5							
Day	A, D, E	A, D, E	A, D, E	A, D, E	A, B, E	B, E	B, E
Night	C	C	C	C	C	D	D

Figure 2.5 demonstrates a second variation of a block schedule using five hospitalists. In this model, four of the five hospitalists are working at any one time (weekdays), and all five providers work some time during each week.

This model eliminates call (e.g., any shift over 12 hours). Compared to a five-hospitalist block schedule (Figure 2.4), this schedule increases the amount of weekend work. Each provider works three out of five weekends, two of which are consecutive. Each hospitalist gets six consecutive days off each five-week cycle.

Continuity is maintained by the long block of day shifts and by bridging the "new" hospitalist onto the day schedule the Friday of the weekend of call.

*Source: **Kenneth G. Simone, DO,** founder and president, Hospitalist and Practice Solutions, Veazie, ME.*

Figure 2.6 Five-hospitalist seven days on/seven days off schedule

Week 1	Mon.	Tues.	Wed.	Thurs.	Fri.	Sat.	Sun.
Day	A, C	A, C	A, C	A, C	A, C	A, C	C, D
Night	E	E	E	E	E	A	C
Week 2							
Day	B, D	B, D	B, D	B, D	B, D	B, D	A, B
Night	E	E	E	E	E	D	B
Week 3							
Day	A, E	A, E	A, E	A, E	A, E	A, E	B, E
Night	C	C	C	C	C	A	E
Week 4							
Day	B, D	B, D	B, D	B, D	B, D	B, D	D, E
Night	C	C	C	C	C	B	D
Week 5							
Day	A, E	A, E	A, E	A, E	A, E	A, E	A, B
Night	D	D	D	D	D	E	A
Week 6							
Day	B, C	B, C	B, C	B, C	B, C	B, C	C, E
Night	D	D	D	D	D	B	C
Week 7							
Day	D, E	D, E	D, E	D, E	D, E	D, E	D, C
Night	A	A	A	A	A	E	D
Week 8							
Day	B, C	B, C	B, C	B, C	B, C	B, C	B, D
Night	A	A	A	A	A	C	B
Week 9							
Day	D, E	D, E	D, E	D, E	D, E	D, E	A, E
Night	B	B	B	B	B	D	E
Week10							
Day	A, C	A, C	A, C	A, C	A, C	A, C	D, C
Night	B	B	B	B	B	A	C
Week 11							
Day	B, D	B, D	B, D	B, D	B, D	B, D	B, C
Night	E	E	E	E	E	D	B
Week 12							
Day	A, C	A, C	A, C	A, C	A, C	A, C	A, B
Night	E	E	E	E	E	C	A
Week 13							
Day	B, D	B, D	B, D	B, D	B, D	B, D	D, E
Night	C	C	C	C	C	B	D
Week 14							
Day	A, E	A, E	A, E	A, E	A, E	A, E	A, B
Night	C	C	C	C	C	E	A

 © 2006 HCPro, Inc. TOOLS AND STRATEGIES FOR AN EFFECTIVE HOSPITALIST PROGRAM

| Figure | 2.6 | Five-hospitalist seven days on/ seven days off schedule (cont.) |

Week 15	Mon.	Tues.	Weds.	Thurs.	Fri.	Sat.	Sun.
Day	B, C	B, C	B, C	B, C	B, C	B, C	A, C
Night	D	D	D	D	D	B	C
Week 16							
Day	A, E	A, E	A, E	A, E	A, E	A, E	C, E
Night	D	D	D	D	D	A	E
Week 17							
Day	B, C	B, C	B, C	B, C	B, C	B, C	B, D
Night	A	A	A	A	A	C	B
Week 18							
Day	D, E	D, E	D, E	D, E	D, E	D, E	C, E
Night	A	A	A	A	A	D	E
Week 19							
Day	A, C	A, C	A, C	A, C	A, C	A, C	A, E
Night	B	B	B	B	B	C	A
Week 20							
Day	D, E	D, E	D, E	D, E	D, E	D, E	A, D
Night	B	B	B	B	B	E	D

Figure 2.6 demonstrates a model where, on average, hospitalists work seven consecutive days, ending their workweek with a 24-hour shift. They then have at least seven days off (unless they work the following week on nights). Continuity is maintained, because at least one hospitalist who worked in a given week has rounds during the weekend shift of that week. All providers work two consecutive weeks of nights (which is defined as Monday through Friday) twice in this 20-week rotation. In total, the hospitalist works eight Saturday and Sunday day shifts, and four Saturday and Sunday night shifts.

The disadvantage of this model is that the clinical director of the hospitalist program is not scheduled to work in the facility every week, and his or her presence is lacking on average every other week. The director may come in on the "off" week, but this will negate the positive aspects of this schedule for him or her.

In addition, because the hospitalists typically work 96 hours in their workweek, they may be less inclined to come in to the hospital on their weeks off to attend meetings or participate in other added-value services (e.g., providing training and education to key hospital personnel). Thus, on average, only half of the hospitalists are in the hospital each week.

If there are six providers working in this model, the sixth provider (typically the clinical director) works Monday through Friday 7 a.m. to 7 p.m., thus establishing administrative presence on a regular basis. The schedule otherwise remains a constant.

*Source: **Kenneth G. Simone, DO,** founder and president, Hospitalist and Practice Solutions, Veazie, ME.*

Figure	2.7	Six-hospitalist seven days on/seven days off schedule

Week 1	Mon.	Tues.	Wed.	Thurs.	Fri.	Sat.	Sun.
Day	A, B	A, B	A, B	A, B	A, B	A, B	D, B
Night	C	C	C	C	C	A	B
Week 2							
Day	D, E	D, E	D, E	D, E	D, E	D, E	C, E
Night	F	F	F	F	F	D	E
Week 3							
Day	A, C	A, C	A, C	A, C	A, C	A, C	A, F
Night	B	B	B	B	B	C	A
Week 4							
Day	D, F	D, F	D, F	D, F	D, F	D, F	B, D
Night	E	E	E	E	E	F	D
Week 5							
Day	B, C	B, C	B, C	B, C	B, C	B, C	C, E
Night	A	A	A	A	A	B	C
Week 6							
Day	E, F	E, F	E, F	E, F	E, F	E, F	A, F
Night	D	D	D	D	D	E	F

Figure 2.7 is a schedule using six hospitalists for a seven days on/seven days off model. This schedule splits the practice into two teams. Hospitalists A, B, and C work together, as do hospitalists D, E, and F (with the exception of the transition over the weekend). This could enhance teamwork, although there is some risk of "splitting" the practice team.

Each hospitalist works seven consecutive days, ending his or her workweek with a 24-hour shift. This is followed by seven consecutive days off. Night call consists of one-week rotations (Monday through Friday), followed by eight days off. This gives the hospitalists sufficient time to get readjusted to days and enjoy their time off. Continuity is maintained, as this schedule provides at least one physician who performs rounds on the weekends who worked during the previous week.

Each hospitalist works two Saturday and two Sunday day shifts, as well as one Saturday and one Sunday night shift in this six-week rotation. As in the five-hospitalist seven days on/seven days off schedule (Figure 2.6), the major disadvantage is that the clinical director of the hospitalist program is scheduled to work only every other week.

Source: **Kenneth G. Simone, DO**, *founder and president, Hospitalist and Practice Solutions, Veazie, ME.*

Adjusting staffing levels using on-call backup

Figure 2.8 demonstrates one facility's method for adjusting staffing to the number of patients or the level of acute patient care required, with the goal of maximizing the use of hospitalists. The checklist within it enables hospitalists to assign patients a "point value" based on patients' acuity. If the total points are equal to or less than 30 on a day when a third physician (i.e., the "float") is scheduled to work from 9:00 a.m. to 9:00 p.m., the float physician is called off from 9:00 a.m. to 3:00 p.m. and instead is placed on call from 3:00 p.m. to 9:00 p.m.

Electronic solutions to scheduling

As the use of technology continues to spread throughout the hospital, it is not surprising that electronic (or Internet-based) physician scheduling systems are gaining in popularity. Advocates say the systems

- save time
- alleviate scheduling conflicts
- better track shift work and time off requests
- help coordinate requests for unique assignments

Figure 2.9 demonstrates one facility's reasoning and process for switching to electronic scheduling.

Figure 2.8 Protocol—Determining the need for on-call backup

Title _____ Hospitalists on call_____

Originating dept._____ Affected dept._____

Vice president approval _____

Chief operating officer approval _____

Original date _____

Revised date _____

Review date _____

Policy: The *(name of hospitalist service)* will use staffing patterns aimed at maximum use of provider resources adjusted to patient census and/or acuity of illness. If a decrease in on-site provider resources is needed, the following will be used to make said adjustments.

Purpose: To facilitate access to the *(name of hospitalist service)* by assuring the availability of adequate resources to meet patients', families', and referring providers' needs while providing safe, efficient quality care.

1. At morning MD TRU Rounds, all patients will be assigned a point value based on acuity. The assigned points are as follows:

   • Critical care   1.5 points

   • Medical/surgical/telemetry   1.0 points

   • Critical care consults   1.5 points

   • Medical/surgical/telemetry consults   1.0 points

2. If the total points are equal to or less than 30 on a day when a third physician (float) is scheduled from 0900 to 2100, the float physician will be called off from 0900 to 1500 and be placed on call from 1500 to 2100.

Figure

2.8   **Protocol—Determining the need for on-call backup (cont.)**

3. When the float physician is reassigned to on call prior to 1500, the point total will be recalculated using 2.0 points for new medical/surgical/telemetry admissions and 2.5 points for all critical care admissions.

4. If the new total is greater than 40, the on call physician will be called in to work the second part of the 0900 to 2100 shift (1500 to 2100).

5. If the new total is equal to or less than 40, the on call physician will be called off for the remainder of the assigned shift.

6. The float physician will not be placed on call on any day that the *(name of hospitalist service)* is scheduled on the emergency department medical unassigned roster.

7. The hospitalist administrator on call will be called prior to any schedule changes.

8. The hospitalist administrator on call will be responsible for ensuring that all schedule changes are recorded on the original time schedule.

*Source: **Jenifir Bruno, MD,** FirstHealth Moore Regional Hospital Hospitalist Service, Pinehurst, NC.*

Figure 2.9 Implementing an electronic, Internet-based solution to scheduling multiple 24/7 shifts involving 30-plus hospitalists across two campuses

Why implement electronic physician scheduling?

The decision to automate the hospitalist schedule (with its various shifts) was not made solely based on the complexity and number of providers. Additional benefits include the ability to

- track scheduled hours

- tally totals

- track trades

- tally hours for any extra payments owed those who have worked beyond their contracted hours

Implementation plan:

One hospitalist has been assigned the role of "lead scheduler" and is given credit hours each month in return. This individual downloads the tool from Spiral Software (*www.spiralsoftware.com*), which has an annual price of $250.00. This fee includes licensing for software, as well as Web posting of the schedule. The schedule, once posted, can be viewed from anywhere via the Internet and modified ad lib by the lead scheduler.

The tool has been of use not only in accurately tracking excess hour payments (e.g., to justify additional budgeted full-time personnel), but also in calculating total rounding days. The latter is used to monitor the efficiency-related metric of discharges per rounding day.

*Source: **Mary Dallas, MD,** and **Revathi A-Davidson, MPH,** Presbyterian Healthcare Services/Presbyterian Hospital, Albuquerque, NM.*

Recruitment

3

Recruitment

Jeffrey R. Dichter, MD, FACP

Recruitment is the most important process for virtually every hospitalist program. It is also labor inten-sive, time consuming, and difficult. The demand for hospitalists is intense, and those practitioners of greatest desirability are relatively scarce. Most programs execute the recruitment process competently, but only a few execute the process extremely well, and their chances of getting the best candidates are the greatest.

This chapter overviews the recruitment process and highlights the most important aspects of recruiting. It complements the recruitment checklist that accompanies it.

Define your program

The first objective in the recruitment process is to define your hospitalist program as thoroughly as pos-sible, identifying the service's key characteristics. This activity has several important consequences:

- Hospitals with well-defined hospitalist programs are better equipped to select hospitalist candi-dates who are most likely to be interested in their programs. Similarly, well-defined programs help candidates "self-select" out if they are not interested in what the program has to offer.
- A well-defined program with a clear vision for the future makes a positive and effective impres-

sion on candidates about program leadership. Candidates are likely to think that the program leaders are competent and that the program is likely to be successful in the future. Well-defined programs also project the conviction that the leadership will follow through on promises and plans that are made during the recruitment process.

- The end result of defining your program should be the ability to spend your resources recruiting candidates who best fit your program type, size, and culture, while minimizing efforts aimed at those who are not likely to be interested.

The hospitalist program characteristics listed in the section below are among the most important that programs should address in the recruitment process.

Characteristics of a hospitalist program practice

The following are examples of the traits that define a hospitalist practice:

- Teaching hospital
- Nonteaching hospital/program
- Large hospital
- Small facility
- Urban setting
- Rural environment
- One or more practice settings, facilities, or hospitals covered by hospitalists
- Workload schedule
    -Call-based versus in-house
    -Amount of time off, and how it is structured and administrated
- Workload characteristics
    -Average daily census
    -Frequency of call
    -Duration of call
    -Typical number of admissions on call
    -Frequency of weekend and night call
- Compensation characteristics
    -Salary

        -Bonus structure

        -Combination

- Career growth opportunities

        -Teaching opportunities

        -Research opportunities

        -Professional advancement, leadership, and entrepreneurial opportunities

- The opportunity to build or participate in new programs
- Medical directorships
- Consultation practices

Other items that will help candidates assess your program include the following:

- The culture, mission, and values of the program
- The key strengths and potential weaknesses of the program
- How the program compares with that of local competitors
- Whether expectations for hospitalists in the program are clearly defined
- Things that make the program unique

        -Key leaders in field affiliated with the program

        -Unique specialty care or specialty programs the service provides

- The plans program leadership has for development and growth during the next one to three years
- Restrictive covenant (noncompete) clauses the program may have

Candidates' observations about hospitalist programs

Every hospitalist program, in addition to having a precise definition of itself, should have a clear sense of how candidates perceive the recruitment process.

Resident trainees and practicing hospitalists are busy physicians with professional and personal responsibilities that demand most of their time. Although the process of searching for employment is as important to them as it is for the programs recruiting them, they have a limited amount of time and personal energy to dedicate to the process.

With the current intense competition for hospitalists' skills and services, hospitalists are often bombarded with job opportunities from multiple avenues, ranging from recruiters to friends. Any prospective program has only a limited chance to catch the attention of good prospective candidates.

Therefore, every interaction with a prospective candidate should be viewed as a precious opportunity. Each contact with a candidate should be planned and executed on time, with a priority placed on the relay of complete and accurate program information. Prompt follow-through is critical.

The following are examples of how to treat candidates, to leave them with positive impressions of your program:

- Treat them with the utmost courtesy and respect
- Provide a prompt follow-up call or contact after the candidate's initial connection with the hospitalist service
- Be friendly, informative, and welcoming during the initial phone interview
- Provide thorough information about the program via a telephone call, a letter, an information packet received by mail, or an e-mail with a link to the program and hospital's Web site
- Make the interview process a positive experience
- Follow through adequately after the interview(s)

Include hospitalists' families in the recruitment process

Hospitalist candidates undoubtedly are focused on exploring the job-related characteristics of prospective programs, including

- compensation and benefits
- history of the program
- program mission, objectives, and values
- hospitalist staff makeup and camaraderie
- medical staff composition and relationship to the hospitalist program
- hospitalists' relationships with the hospital administration

However, consider that the decision-making process typically includes other individuals associated with the candidate and that factors other than those listed above may contribute to successfully closing the deal. As a result, recruitment should be equally directed toward the candidate's significant other and/or family, if applicable.

To recruite in this way, incorporate information about the community, such as what is shown in the following list, as it might affect a candidate's decision to move or transfer to the region:

- Neighborhoods
- School systems
- Safety
- Population and growth estimates
- Major industries
- Taxes
- Extracurricular activities (e.g., sports teams, beaches, mountains, etc.)
- Cultural opportunities
- Neighboring communities

Detailed disclosure about the community may help eliminate the culture shock that often accompanies relocation. This is especially true for the hospitalist's significant other and family. Often, a hiring mismatch occurs due to the unmet expectations of someone other than the candidate.

The recruitment process and the recruitment checklist

The recruitment process may be divided into three primary segments:

1. Finding and assessing hospitalist candidates
2. The interview process
3. Follow-up and follow-through to closure

Figure 3.1 is a recruitment checklist that further defines these three areas of the recruitment process and enables programs to build a new recruitment plan or add-on to an existing one. The steps outlined in the checklist are a list of the key items and issues that all programs should address in defining the recruitment process. It is not intended to be an all-inclusive list, and all steps may not apply or be necessary for every program.

Figure	3.1	The recruitment checklist

1. Finding and assessing hospitalist candidates

   • **List the places where you can gather potential candidates' curricula vitae (CV)**

   - Recruiters (in-house or third-party)

   - Advertisements in medical society or other publications

   - Web sites

   - Organizations' teaching programs

   - Word of mouth (e.g., staff hospitalists or other professionals affiliated with your program)

   - Other sources

   • **Determine what will occur when potential candidates are identified**

   - Decide how quickly your program will review CVs and determine how to initiate contact with desirable candidates

      • No more than 48 hours *(recommended standard)*

   -Assign an individual to review incoming CVs

      • Program director or designee

      • Practice administrator

      • Other

   - Decide which individual will make the initial contact with the candidate, and assess whether more than one individual will participate at this stage

      • Practice administrator

      • Program director or designee

      • Some combination of program representatives

      • Other

   - Determine how the initial contact with the candidate will be made

      • Phone call *(strongly recommended)*

      • E-mail

      • Other

   - After the initial contact, decide whether to pursue the candidate

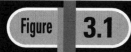

The recruitment checklist (cont.)

- Define how this decision will be made and determine which individual will have the final say
    - Usually made by the hospitalist program director or designee and/or practice administrator
    - Determine the method by which desirable candidates will be notified of the program's interest and invited for an on-site interview
- At the time of initial contact
- Afterward
    - Via telephone call *(recommended)*
    - E-mail or letter *(less personal and not recommended in most circumstances)*
    - Decide whether and how candidates who are not chosen for interviews will be notified
- Inform candidate he or she is not being pursued as a candidate *(recommended)*
    - Discuss whether an information packet or e-mail will be sent to desirable candidates after the initial contact
- Send an "interview invitation" with pertinent information *(strongly recommended)*
- Consider sending additional information to desirable candidates
    - Information packet
    - Video or DVD describing the hospitalist program, the hospital, and other important information
    - Other

2. The interview process
  - **Determine how the interviews will be arranged**

  - Define responsibilities:
    - Assign a key contact person who will interact regularly with the candidate *(strongly recommended)*
        - This will be the "go to" person whom the candidates will contact for all needs that they may have during the interview process and subsequent stages up to acceptance
    - Designate one person who is responsible for the coordination of the interview.
        - This is usually the key contact person, but it can be someone else
    - Determine the key contact person's responsibilities:

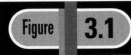

The recruitment checklist (cont.)

-Coordinate potential interview or call dates on candidate's and program's calendars

-Arrange an interview schedule for the candidate's visit

-Ensure that all involved parties remain on schedule the day of the interview, and be prepared for changes routinely made at the last minute (see "Develop contingency plans for changing the interview schedule at the last minute")

-Assist the candidate in making arrangements, such as booking an airline flight, a rental car, and hotel accommodations (as needed), as well as in getting directions or making other visit arrangements

-Decide whether the candidate will be reimbursed for expenses

• What expenses are to be reimbursed?

-Airline tickets, hotel room, rental car *(strongly recommended)*

-Meals

-Other expenses

• Determine how the expenses are to be handled/reimbursed

-Reimbursement after receipts are received from candidate.

-Key expenses paid for up-front by program.

-Other mechanisms.

-Clearly define (in writing) for the candidate how, when, and for what expenses he or she will be reimbursed. Send this information to the candidate as part of the interview invitation *(recommended).*

• **Decide how the interview will be conducted**

- Determine which individual will be responsible for the candidate at all times while he or she is on site

• This is often the person who is responsible for coordinating the interview process

• If multiple individuals are designated, clearly define each person's specific responsibilities:

-Interview the candidate

-Ensure that the candidate is where he or she should be, and with whom, at designated times

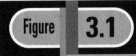

Figure 3.1   **The recruitment checklist (cont.)**

-Ensure that the candidate's other needs (e.g., meals, restroom access, other) are met

-Determine which individuals the candidate will meet

- Program director

- Practice administrator and staff

- Hospital administrator

- Staff hospitalists

- Case mangers, nurses, or other hospital personnel

- Others

-Distribute to all interviewers (ahead of time):

- The candidate's CV

- A copy of the full day's schedule

- Any other pertinent information

-Outline any other key events that will be scheduled for candidates

- Tour of hospital, practice, other places

- Discussion of business issues

-Personnel who are knowledgeable and skilled at speaking about these issues should fulfill this role

- Social event: typically lunch and/or dinner

-Map out the conclusion of the interview

- Conduct a formal wrap-up with the candidate, typically with the program director or practice administrator *(strongly recommended)*

    -Wrap-up provides the candidate with an opportunity to ask questions at the end of interview and enables program personnel to receive feedback from the candidate

    -Schedule a formal follow-up post interview (strongly recommended)

        o This part of the process should be shared with the candidate during the interview or at its conclusion

        o This is typically a phone call *(recommended)* or other communication in a defined time interval *(two weeks or less recommended)*

        o Follow-up communication should be initiated by program personnel, usually the program director or designee, or the practice administrator

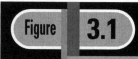

The recruitment checklist (cont.)

-Develop contingency plans for changing the interview schedule at the last minute, as the clinical demands of virtually every practice will necessitate this

• Most candidates expect this

• Candidates are likely to be favorably impressed by programs that manage this well

3. Follow-up and follow-through to closure

• **Outline a procedure for post interview follow-up**

-Schedule prompt feedback meetings with all personnel who interviewed the candidate *(strongly recommended)*

• Decide whether personnel who interviewed the candidate will return verbal or written feedback on the candidate, typically within 48 hours

-Decide how the decision about the desirability of the candidate will be made

• Typically by the program director and/or practice administrator after receiving feedback from all participants in the interview process

• Decisions should be shared with all staff hospitalists after they are made

-Create a three-tiered system for determining the desirability of candidates *(recommended)*

• Candidates who are definitely wanted

• Candidates who are acceptable second choices

• Candidates who are not desired

-Schedule contact with candidates

• Disposition completed on schedule (see above)

• Position offered: Yes or No

• Candidate accepts: Yes or No

-Solicit references for candidates who are offered a position and who are seriously interested

• May consist of a simple phone call to references or formal written letters, as appropriate for your program

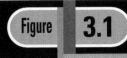

The recruitment checklist (cont.)

• Determine how formal offers of employment will be made

-Send a formal letter of acceptance

• Include a contract if necessary *(recommended)*

-Set a date by which the candidate should respond to the offer

• Typically two to three weeks

-Determine whether legal counsel should prepare or review the contract *(recommended)*

• Note that dealing with legal counsel can be time-consuming; therefore, a time

frame for this should be clearly defined and factored into the overall process

When your hospitalist program's interview process is fully developed, create a timetable for each step and for the overall process. Although the timetable will vary somewhat with each candidate, it is helpful in systematically tracking progress. Good luck!

Source: **Jeffrey R. Dichter, MD, FACP,** *previous president, Society of Hospital Medicine; partner, Medical Consultants PC, Muncie, IN; founder, Hospital Medicine Program at Ball Memorial Hospital, Muncie, IN; and practicing hospitalist and internist.*

Retention
and orientation

4

Retention and orientation

Kenneth G. Simone, DO

Jeffrey R. Dichter, MD, FACP

The job postings sections of hospitalist-targeted publications provide ample anecdotal evidence that the demand for these professionals outweighs the supply.

However, it's the hard numbers from the Society of Hospital Medicine (*www.hospitalmedicine.org*) and a growing cache of studies that prove that the proliferation of hospital medicine programs is stretching thin the supply of hospitalists nationwide.[1]

As a result, retention should be foremost—whether your hospitalist program is well established or just getting on its feet. To reduce turnover, consider investing in a formal, standardized retention program that involves participation by medical staff leaders and hospitalists on staff. Consider ways to make retention a part of the organization's culture, rather than a stand-alone goal.

Retention starts in the job interview

You might be surprised to learn that the retention process actually begins during a hospitalist candidate's first interview. Most physicians who leave their organization do so in the first five years, and often the decision to leave occurs within the first three to five months of employment.[2]

> **Initial interview guidelines**
>
> - Set clear expectations about compensation and long-term goals, clinical performance, and quality standards
> - Provide realistic details about the culture of your hospitalist program, hospital, and health system
> - Seek feedback on the candidate's expectations and desires
> - Objectively evaluate the match

Question candidates with retention in mind

Successful recruiters know that employee retention begins long before a candidate is hired. A particular strength of hospitalist programs that are successful in keeping great hospitalists on staff is their adeptness at monitoring the warning signs a candidate's comments and questions portray during the interview process. If all of a candidate's questions are about compensation and vacation, it should be viewed as a red flag.

> The following are examples of the inquiries you should hear from hospitalist candidates during the interview process:
>
> - What are the physicians in the group like?
> - How long have they been there?
> - What is the rate of turnover?
> - What are the group dynamics like?
> - What is the diversity of cases I can expect?
> - What's the average patient population?
> - What is the on-call scheduling model?

Your questions for candidates that keep retention in the foreground include the following:

- Why are you thinking about making a move?
- What's important to you in your career?
- Why are you interested in being a hospitalist?
- What are your subspecialty interests?
- What is your preference for scheduling?
- How flexible are you in terms or coverage hours/scheduling?
- Would you be opposed to working nights?
- Why have you chosen to interview at this program, and what other programs are you looking at?
- What are your long-term goals?
- What are your professional aspirations?

Remember: In the face of physician shortages and increased patient demand, it can be difficult to objectively evaluate issues such as fit and long-term expectations. However, securing the right hospitalists up front will help save your facility time and money in the long run.

Survey new hospitalists

One method of ensuring that a new hospitalist is receiving the assistance and feedback he or she needs is to conduct a brief survey six to 10 weeks after the physician's start date. Doing so will ensure that the program is keeping its word in terms of fulfilling the expectations set forth in the interview.

More importantly, the practice of surveying new hospitalists can help stem the problem of turnover because it gives new staff a formal outlet for addressing any potential problems before the issues explode and cause them to resign. (It's perfectly appropriate to ask outright: Is there anything you are experiencing that would cause you to think about leaving?) Finally, soliciting comments—both positive and negative—from hospitalists new to the program shows an interest in the hospitalist's progress and professional growth.

Figure 4.1 is a sample form for surveying new hospitalists. This form may be administered to the new hospitalists by the hospitalist program director, medical director, or other appropriate medical staff leader in a one-on-one meeting approximately six to 10 weeks after the physician's start date. In addition to reviewing practice reports with the new hospitalist at this time, the administrator can ask specific questions about his or her experience during orientation and record any feedback about areas to improve.

Employ a comprehensive orientation program

A comprehensive orientation program should be a large part of your retention efforts. After all, your program has already completed the difficult tasks of poring over countless curricula vitae and selecting and hiring the best hospitalists.

It's time to ensure that, once on the job, hospitalists have the tools and support they need to perform successfully in their clinical and other medical leadership roles. In fact, hospitals that simply welcome the new hospitalist and then leave him or her stranded with minimal assistance are asking for disaster.

After hiring hospitalists, an appropriate transition into their roles is critical to ensuring a solid, successful organization with a stable work force. In addition, because success as a hospitalist requires skills that are not covered in a residency program, a structured approach to orientation and training is essential.

Cover at least the following during a hospitalist's orientation:

- An explanation of your practice model and key operating principles
- An overview of the materials provided in the job expectations policy
- Practice structure and relationships
- Documentation standards
- Report and sign-out processes
- Communication standards
- Processes for follow-up care and handoffs
- Discussion of the organization's/hospitalist service's mission, objectives, and values

The orientation process is complemented by the creation and review of a practice and policy procedure manual for hospitalists.

When executed successfully, an orientation program helps foster shared operational expectations among all parties involved in executing the hospitalist program's services.

Figure 4.1 | **New physician retention interview**

Physician: _____ Start Date: _____

Practice Partner: _____ Resource Doc: _____

Interview Date: _____ Medical Director: _____

Signature: _____

A. Performance Data Summary:

   1. Web Reports:

     • Encounters/profitability: ❑ No issues   ❑ Issues identified

       Comments:_____

     • Days to Synch Report: ❑ No issues   ❑ Issues identified

       Comments:_____

     • D/C Compliance Report: ❑ No issues   ❑ Issues identified

       Comments:_____

     • D/C Notification & Samples: ❑ No issues   ❑ Issues identified

       Comments:_____

     • Review LOS (<65 or >65):   ❑ No issues   ❑ Issues identified

       Comments:_____

     • Review Call Center: ❑ No issues   ❑ Issues identified

       Comments:_____

   2. Review Dashboard: ❑ Acceptable   ❑ Issues Noted

   3. Review Standing Orders: ❑ Acceptable   ❑ Issues Noted

   4. Review Expectations: ❑ Acceptable   ❑ Issues Noted

   5. Revenue/Encounter: ❑ Acceptable   ❑ Issues Noted

B. Mentee Feedback:

   1. How do we compare with what we said in your interviewing process?

_____

_____

_____

| Figure 4.1 | New physician retention interview (cont.) |

2. What is working well?

_____

_____

3. How are you handling the transition to being a (name of hospitalist program) hospitalist?

_____

_____

4. Which individuals have been most helpful to you?

_____

_____

5. What systems or ideas do you feel could improve our operations?

_____

_____

6. Is there anything you are experiencing that would cause you to think about leaving?

_____

_____

C. Recommendations/comments for new physicians:

_____

_____

D. Follow-up for medical directors or others:

_____

_____

Source: **_Mary Jo Gorman, MD, MBA,_** _chief medical officer, IPC–The Hospitalist Company._

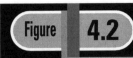

Orientation—Day #1

Regional Office Orientation Checklist

Executive Director	Business Development/Office Manager

1. Meet and greet the new provider.
 	
2. Introduce the hub office staff:
  a) Business development
  b) Credentialing
  c) Office manager
  d) Receptionist
 	
3. Review (name of hospital) videos/DVDs and complete the hospitalist exercise.
  • "What is a hospitalist?" (video) and exercise
  • View retreat DVD
 	
4. Set guidelines for productivity:
  a) Billing and compliance
  b) Encounter goal
  c) Work schedule and image
  d) Timely completion of medical records
 	
5. Present your expectations of a hospitalist:
  a) Practice group and region meetings (time/location)
  b) Leadership retreats
  c) SHM/ACP meetings
  d) Marketing/region strategy
  e) Customer service
 	
6. Distribute the orientation manual and discuss the overall program and schedule for the week:
  a) Assignment of Resource Doctor Mentor
  b) Assignment of Practice Partner
  c) Market and/or client orientation activities, etc.
 	
7. Provide and review the human resources manual
	1. Provide working materials:
	  a) Building access
	  b) Name badge
	  c) Business cards
	  d) Cell phone
	  e) Lab coats
	  f) Pager
	
	2. Conduct document review:
	  a) Hospital privileges
	  b) Medicare and Medicaid applications
	  c) Malpractice insurance applications
	  d) Photograph and biography for Web site
	  e) Employee data sheet
	  f) W-4 form; other HR forms
	  g) Direct deposit application
	  h) Benefits package (dental, medical, etc.)
	
	3. Present and explain:
	  a) Call schedule for the practice group
	  b) Human resources policies for vacation, CME, sick time, etc.
	  c) Orientation to answering service and/or training as needed
	
	4. Ensure attendance at billing training.
	
	5. Ensure that the provider has the orientation schedule for the balance of the week, including the schedule for the Resource Doctor Mentor

*Source: **Mary Jo Gorman, MD, MBA,** chief medical officer, IPC–The Hospitalist Company.*

Figure 4.3   Orientation—Day #4

Hospital Tour Checklist & Consultant Resource List

Hospital tour checklist Department/functions:	Consultants Hospital #1 Name:	Consultants Hospital #2 Name:
☐ Emergency Dept: Director, Patient Board, Physicians	Cardiology: _____ _____	Cardiology: _____ _____
☐ Professional Staff/Physician Services Office	Pulmonary & CC: _____ _____	Pulmonary & CC: _____ _____
☐ Case Management & Social Services Dept.	GI: _____	GI: _____
☐ Nursing Management/VP of Nursing	Gen. Surgery: _____	Gen. Surgery: _____
☐ ICU/CCU	Ortho: _____	Ortho: _____

☐ Nursing Units:
    Tele/Med Surg
    Sub Acute/Rehab
    Day Surg/Short Stay
    Others, as appropriate
	Neurology: _____ _____	Neurology: _____ _____

☐ Cafeteria/Phys. Dining Room ☐ Med Records/Transcription ☐ IT Department (Computer Codes) ☐ Security/Doctor's Parking ☐ Switchboard Operators	Neurosurgery: _____ _____ Hem/Oncology: _____	Neurosurgery: _____ _____ Hem/Oncology: _____
☐ Radiology (Dictation Line)	Nephrology: _____ _____	Nephrology: _____ _____

☐ Ancillary Support
  ☐ EKG & ECHO
  ☐ Hemodialysis Unit
  ☐ Lab & Micro
  ☐ Blood Bank
	Urology: _____ _____	Urology: _____ _____

☐ Hospital Library	ID: _____ _____	ID: _____ _____
☐ Pastoral Service		

☐ Services Unavailable:
  ☐ No MRI
  ☐ No Cath
  ☐ No Consultants
☐ Surgeries unable to perform
	<u>Identified PCP partners</u> for outpatient follow-up:
	
	_____
	_____
		<u>Identified PCP partners</u> for outpatient follow-up:
		
		_____
		_____

Additional Notes:

Source: **Mary Jo Gorman, MD, MBA,** *chief medical officer, IPC–The Hospitalist Company*

 © 2006 HCPRO, INC. TOOLS AND STRATEGIES FOR AN EFFECTIVE HOSPITALIST PROGRAM

Tailoring the orientation style or duration to individual hospitalists is good practice, when possible. For example, an experienced hospitalist may be ready to assume his or her role after just three days of orientation, whereas a physician transitioning from a residency program may require five or more days of orientation.

Make sure that you are covering all of the bases in your orientation program: Use comprehensive check-lists detailing new hospitalists' first days on the job. They should be specific, down to the detail of naming the individual who will tour the new physician through the facility on day one, for example.

Figures 4.2 and 4.3 are sample checklists for orientation days one and four, used primarily to ensure that pertinent information is covered with the new hospitalist.

Use physicians on staff as mentors

When it comes to the key items new hospitalists need to know to succeed in your organization, no one on the medical staff knows better than your current hospitalists. Consider giving them a large role in a new hospitalist's first weeks on the job, in addition to having them do the typical rounds with new staff hospitalists.

Mentoring also plays an important role in a hospitalist program's success. Carefully select a mentor for each new hospitalist—that person will help determine the overall success of the orientation experience. To facilitate a strong match, gather information about the new hospitalist and pair him or her with a mentor who shares a similar personality, background, work style, etc.

Finally, consider training your hospitalist mentors. This need not require a large time investment on the part of the mentor. It may entail simply orienting him or her about the standard issues to cover and providing a checklist of items that should be covered during the orientation period.

The orientation program mentor should regularly check in with his or her mentee for at least the first six months and help the new hire (and significant other/family) integrate into the program, hospital, and community.

References

1. Hoangmai H. Pham, MD; Kelly J. Devers, PhD; Sylvia Kuo, PhD; Robert Berenson, MD; "Health Care Market Trends and the Evolution of Hospitalist Use and Roles," *Journal of General Internal Medicine 20*, 20, no. 2 (February 2005): 101–107.

2. Paul Smallwood, "Recruiting tip of the month: How to retain great hospitalists," *Hospitalist Management Advisor* 2, no. 2 (February 2006): 8.

The referring
provider's perspective

5

The referring provider's perspective

Kenneth G. Simone, DO

Providers that refer patients to a hospitalist program vary widely in professional degrees and specialty training. They may be physician assistants (PA); nurse practitioners (NP); primary care physicians (PCP), such as family practitioners, internists, pediatricians, obstetrician/gynecologists; or specialists of various types. They may be outpatient-based (e.g., PCPs) or work within the hospital (e.g., specialists). As a result, each enters into a working relationship with the hospitalist with drastically different expectations. The hospitalist must be sensitive to this fact to make the experience successful for the patient and his or her family, the referring provider, and the hospitalist.

Referring providers' expectations

In most instances, the referring provider views the hospitalist as an extension of his or her medical practice—in other words, a hospital-based partner—and views the hospitalist service as a complement to the outpatient care rendered. As partners in the delivery of healthcare, there is a presumed collegial respect and a desire for open communication. Many expectations are inherent in such a working arrangement. Preferably, to foster a successful relationship, the clinical director of the hospitalist program will meet with the referring provider at the onset of his or her partnership with the hospitalist service to discuss expectations and scope of services.

Understanding the daily responsibilities of providers

To understand the perspective of the referring provider, hospitalists must gain an appreciation for what transpires during his or her "typical" day. The myriad pressures a provider encounters daily include

- caring for many patients in need of acute and chronic care
- providing preventative care
- reviewing laboratory and clinical studies
- coordinating appropriate follow-up care within a larger healthcare network
- corresponding with patients' families
- managing aspects of the staff and business office
- interacting with specialists and hospitalist providers

In addition, referring providers face numerous insurance-related tasks. These include developing an intimate working knowledge of each company's medication formulary (in most instances, the insurer offers multiple products and, thus, multiple formularies) and specialty network. Providers must balance this information with what they feel is in the best medical interest of patients.

Superimposed on these responsibilities is the need to consider the cost of patient care, including what fees will be passed on to the patient. Voluminous paperwork accompanies the referral and prior authorization process for many "controlled" studies (e.g., magnetic resonance imaging studies and computed tomography scans) and medications.

Considering the many pressures and responsibilities encountered in modern medicine, it is little wonder that the referring provider requires an efficient, effective, and informative hospitalist program with which to partner. Hospitalists must be sensitive to the demands placed on referring providers and work within their system to strengthen the physician/patient relationship. This entails having an appreciation and respect for the long-term relationship that has developed between the PCP and patient.

What providers expect from hospitalists

At a minimum, a referring provider expects the hospitalist to provide notification on admission of his or her patient to the hospital, updates that include any acute changes in patient status, and notification of patient discharge. Daily correspondence by voicemail, fax, e-mail, or other means (e.g., transmission of electronic record) would be a premium. Timely delivery of the patient's history and physical, discharge summary, and pertinent laboratory results/studies is essential.

What hospitalists can expect in return

In return, referring providers should ensure that the hospitalist receives valuable patient data, including the following:

- Information about the patient's current problem
- The patient's medication and allergy list
- Pertinent clinical and laboratory studies
- The do-not-resuscitate status of the patient
- Next-of-kin information
- Past medical history

The referring provider should also share with the hospitalist any other information thought to be useful, such as a patient's psychosocial issues, family dynamics, problem-patient issues, and suggestions on how aggressively to treat or work up a patient. Finally, he or she should be available for consultation with the hospitalist in case any unforeseen issues arise.

Understanding the daily responsibilities of specialists

The specialist as a referring provider has his or her own set of expectations and considerations when using a hospitalist service. Specialists typically see patients in the hospital, and many perform hospital-based procedures. Their typical days may be divided between the office and hospital (or multiple hospital sites). They may dedicate certain days in the hospital to perform surgery or other procedures (e.g., colonoscopy, bronchoscopy, coronary angiography, lithotripsy). The specialist may call upon the hospitalist for an urgent consultation to clear a patient for a procedure.

In addition to these day-to-day responsibilities, specialists are not exempt from completing office and hospital paperwork, including patients' progress and procedure notes and insurance forms. Many specialists also maintain hospital staff leadership posts and fulfill hospital committee obligations.

How specialists view hospitalists

The acceptance of hospitalists by specialists is divided. Some see hospitalists as competitors who may take consultations away. Others appreciate the hospitalists' role and have an interest in using them as an extension of their practice. In general, most specialists acknowledge the accessibility of the hospitalist and the ease with which a "curbside" or official consultation can be obtained. In any case, it is the responsibility of hospitalists to educate and advocate for their specialt, and to take an active role in building relationships with specialists.

Many specialists express a desire to transition from direct inpatient care to a consultant role. In this scenario, they would consult and make clinical recommendations without being involved in the daily management of the patient. This relationship may alleviate the endless hospital work (e.g., performing histories and physicals, dictating discharge summaries, providing daily hospital rounds/notes, and dealing with utilization review and insurer issues) with which they are saddled. Changing roles would enable the specialist to become a "procedurist" (a term coined by Kenneth G. Simone, DO, for physicians who dedicate the majority of their time to performing various procedures in their field of expertise—i.e., a procedure-oriented professional). Procedurists provide hospital care on an as-needed basis. This arrangement presents an opportunity for a symbiotic professional relationship between hospitalist and specialist.

Figure 5.1 and **Figure 5.2** represent the "wish lists" of referring providers and specialists with regard to their expectations about using a hospitalist service.

Figure 5.1   **The referring provider's 'wish list' for hospitalist services**

- Hospitalist practice/patient education pamphlets for the provider's office
- Users' manual for the hospitalist services
- Ease of access to the hospitalist
- Notification of the provider at the time of his or her patient's admission
- Communication at expected times (e.g., admission, significant changes in medical status, discharge, death)
- Real-time delivery of important hospital paperwork
- Coordination of care (e.g., no duplication of studies)
- Teamwork and respect for the longstanding patient/primary care physician outpatient relationship (act as "partners" and do not undermine the outpatient care administered)
- Coordination of the outpatient follow-up plan
- Medication reconciliation at discharge with sensitivity to the patient's medication formulary
- Continuity at readmission (e.g., if possible, the same hospitalist cares for the patient when he or she is readmitted)

Source: ***Kenneth G. Simone, DO,*** *founder and president, Hospitalist and Practice Solutions, Veazie, ME.*

Figure 5.2   **The specialist's 'wish list' for hospitalist services**

- Ease of access to the hospitalist (e.g., for consultation or to assume care)
- Continued utilization of (consultation with) their specialty services by the hospitalist program
- Greater emphasis on the specialist as consultant, rather than the physician of record
- Communication at standardized, expected times (e.g., admission, significant changes in medical status, discharge, death)
- Real-time delivery of important hospital paperwork
- Coordination of the outpatient follow-up plan

Source: ***Kenneth G. Simone, DO,*** *founder and president, Hospitalist and Practice Solutions, Veazie, ME.*

Communication with healthcare practitioners

6

Communication with healthcare practitioners

Kenneth G. Simone, DO

Communication is an essential component of a successful hospitalist program. It separates an informal coverage arrangement from an integrated healthcare delivery system. A hospitalist must possess the clinical acumen to ensure a successful clinical outcome in the hospital, whereas hospitalist program must employ a comprehensive communication system to deliver a successful service across the healthcare network.

Success is defined as maintaining continuity of care while minimizing the "voltage drop," avoiding the "fumble," streamlining the "handoff" process, and being sensitive to and neutralizing the "black hole."

Hospitalist-related nomenclature

Voltage drop: the loss of information across the hospital threshold (a term coined by **Robert Wachter, MD**, professor of medicine at the University of California, San Francisco Medical Center)

Handoff: the transfer of patient care between providers

Fumble: the mishandling or loss of patient information

Black hole: the time from a patient's hospital discharge until his or her first appointment with the primary care physician (PCP)

Procedurists: physicians who dedicate the majority of their time to performing various procedures in their fields of expertise—procedure-oriented professionals (a term coined by **Kenneth G. Simone, DO**)

Communication modalities

Information exchange between providers can occur in many ways, including telephone, fax, e-mail, voicemail, and electronic medical record. At a minimum, data transferred between the referring physician and the hospitalist should include

- a notification of the patient's admission
- a copy of the patient's history and physical (H&P) evaluation
- any clinical updates
- a copy of the patient's discharge summary

This information must be delivered in an expedient manner. To maintain consistency, use standardized templates for the H&P and discharge summary, and follow standard protocol for contacting referring physicians. The advantages of requiring all hospitalists in the program to use the same templates and protocol are consistency of care and comprehensive communication among all participants (i.e., patient, PCP, hospitalist).

Communication between hospitalists and referring physicians is not the only exchange that warrants a closer look, however. The daily relay of information between hospitalists and specialists or other healthcare professionals (e.g., nurses, social workers, discharge planners, physical and occupational therapists) is vital to the efficient delivery of medical care in the hospital. During hospitalization, patients and their families depend on regular updates from hospitalists regarding their clinical status and discharge plan. Upon discharge, a follow-up telephone call within 48 hours from the hospitalist can be valuable to patients in

- answering any questions they may have
- ensuring that they are functioning well at home
- ensuring that they have received their medications and made any necessary follow-up appointments

Follow-up calls from a hospitalist program representative or case manager are acceptable, but a call from the hospitalist carries more weight. In addition to being a good patient safety and marketing tool, a post-discharge call reinforces the hospitalist's discharge plan.

Finally, consider the importance of communication to patients and PCPs about the hospitalist program itself (for more information on this topic, see Chapter 7). Long before an acute, anxiety-provoking episode requiring hospitalization occurs, patients should be made aware that their PCP will "hand over" their care to a hospitalist. This can be accomplished with patient education brochures distributed in referring providers' offices, in the emergency department, and on the hospital wards. A hospitalist program also may consider creating a Web site that describes the service and its location, introduces the participating hospitalists, and details the practice's philosophy.

Below, the advantages and disadvantages of the primary modes of communication that hospitalists use to communicate with providers are outlined.

- **Telephone**

Advantages:

-Enables "real-time" interaction

-Is amenable to in-depth discussions

-Provides collegial interface between providers

Disadvantages:

-May decrease efficiency by disrupting patient flow (pulls the referring physician from the
exam room and pulls the hospitalist off the floor or out of a patient's exam room)

-Busy telephone lines may be a hindrance

• **Voicemail**

Advantages:

-Is easily accessible for both hospitalists and PCPs

-Providers often prefer it

-Is non-intrusive (providers can check in at their own convenience)

Disadvantages:

-Fosters loss of direct collegial contact

-May contribute to loss of information

-HIPAA considerations (the Health Insurance Portability and Accountability Act monitors
the privacy and security of patient information and requires organizations to maintain
documentation for a minimum of six years)

• **Fax**

Advantages:

-Provides provider a direct copy of the record, discharge summary, etc.

-Leaves a paper trail

Disadvantages:

-HIPAA considerations

-Blocked transmission may be a hindrance

-Misdirection (to the wrong provider) may occur, jeopardizing patient privacy

• **E-mail**

Advantages:

-Is easy and convenient for both hospitalists and PCPs

-Is readily accessible in most offices

-Does not require an intermediary (i.e., office staff member)

Disadvantages:

-HIPAA considerations

-Lacks the "human touch"

- **Electronic medical record (EMR)**

Advantages:

-Provides excellent access for both hospitalists and PCPs

-Fosters decreased redundancy in reports

Disadvantages:

-May cause a "voltage drop" when the system is down

-Decreases efficiency in terms of the time it takes to enter data

-Lacks the "human touch"

The communication interface

Hospitalists should be aware of three key points of information exchange that require special attention:

- Admission
- Hospitalization
- Discharge

Admission

At the time of admission or the next business day (for night admissions), the hospitalist should inform the referring provider that his or her patient was admitted, and provide a diagnosis and prognosis. The referring provider can confirm that the individual is their patient and exchange pertinent information. This is known as "the handoff," which is a vital component of maintaining continuity of care.

Information at admission

At a minimum, the referring physician should supply the following information to the hospitalist at the time of admission:

- A brief history of the patient's present illness
- Appropriate labs or outpatient studies
- Patient's medical and surgical history, including any comorbid conditions
- Current medications
- Any medication allergies
- Legal next of kin
- Where appropriate, patient's do-not-resuscitate (DNR) status, living will information, and organ donor status
- Discharge/transfer summary (when appropriate)

Establishing appropriate and effective communication with patients and families from the outset is imperative to the success of any hospitalist program. Communication with the patient and family at admission should address the hospitalist's admission diagnosis, treatment plan, and prognosis, as well as confirm the patient's DNR status. The hospitalist should assure the family at admission that he or she will be in close communication with the patient's PCP throughout the hospitalization. This also may be an opportune time for the hospitalist to identify the family "spokesperson," solicit questions from the patient and significant others, and distribute a patient education brochure that describes the hospitalist service.

> The following checklist outlines the minimum information that a hospitalist should discuss with a patient and family at the point of admission:
>
> ____ Admission diagnosis
>
> ____ Treatment plan
>
> ____ Prognosis
>
> ____ Expected hospital course
>
> ____ DNR status
>
> ____ Identity of the family spokesperson
>
> ____ Receipt of the hospitalist practice brochure, other literature
>
> ____ Confirmation of PCP

Another consideration during the admission process is ensuring that the hospitalist has clear and concise communication with key hospital personnel. It is essential to involve sub-specialists and ancillary hospital staff—as well as staff from nursing, social services, and utilization management departments, as appropriate–during admission. This may be accomplished in person, via telephone, in the admission orders, and in the H&P. Notably, plans are initiated at admission both for the acute care of the patient and for his or her anticipated discharge. It can be argued that—more than any other time—hospitalists' communication, organizational, and leadership skills are most prominently on display during the admission process.

The following listing shows standard items on an H&P form used at admission:

1. Name of PCP
2. Chief complaint
3. History of present illness (narrative of symptoms that led to the patient's admission)
4. Patient's past medical history
5. Patient's past surgical history
6. Medicine allergies
7. Current medications/immunizations
8. Patient's social history
   - Habits
   - Occupational history
9. Patient's family history
10. Review of systems
11. Physical examination
    - Pelvic examination if relevant to history
    - Rectal examination if indicated
12. Clinical data available (e.g., lab, x-ray, electrocardiogram, etc).
13. Impressions
    - List all active problems identified
    - List all past history
    - List allergies
14. Plan of care
    - Brief outline of management plan
    - Do not resuscitate status
    - Identification of family spokesperson

Hospitalization

The hospitalist must remain in continuous contact with the treatment team during a patient's hospitalization. This can be accomplished through the use of interdisciplinary morning rounds that involve appropriate nursing staff, social services, discharge planners, physical/occupation therapists, and pharmacy staff. Hold these rounds early in the morning so that the day can be dedicated to accomplishing the goals set forth in this meeting.

Preferably, the hospitalist will evaluate the patient twice daily. The afternoon rounds serve to assess the patient's response to the morning treatment plan and therapy, and to make any necessary adjustments. This contributes to the decrease in length of stay, improved efficiency, and cost effectiveness seen in many hospitalist programs. Family conferences also may occur at this time.

The hospitalist must converse with any consultant involved in the case to clearly define that practitioner's role in the patient's care. The hospitalists will also need to speak with various "procedurists" or subspecialists (e.g., radiologists, cardiologists, etc.) to discuss the results of the studies performed. The hospitalist also may contact the referring physician by voicemail, e-mail, fax, or telephone to provide an update. Such communication between providers is essential to the success of the hospitalist service.

If the hospitalist is going off-service, it is important that an off-service note be written to inform both the provider who is assuming care and all other hospital personnel involved in the delivery of care to the patient that a transfer of care has occurred.

The following sample disposition includes the information a hospitalist should report when going off-service:

Use "subjective, objective, assessment, plan (SOAP)" format for chart notes and list

- all medications the patient is taking
- diet
- activity level
- PCP
- DNR status
- brief hospital course to date with pertinent findings

Discharge

The discharge process poses multiple challenges for the hospitalist and the healthcare network. The patient and his or her final outcome may be the most vulnerable at this time (i.e., the "black hole"). Communication is essential to ensure continuity of care and a successful post-hospital course for the patient. It is imperative for the hospitalist to accurately identify where and to whom the discharge information flows. Note that there are instances when multiple individuals and facilities must receive discharge information.

If a patient is discharged directly home, a home health nurse, physical or occupational therapist, or hospice services practitioner may assist him or her there. Thus the appropriate agencies must receive the patient's discharge information.

On the other hand, a patient may be discharged to a rehabilitation facility such as a skilled nursing facility, a boarding home, or a long-term-care facility. In many instances, the attending provider will differ from the patient's referring physician or PCP. As a result, all providers involved in the patient's care must receive a copy of the patient's discharge summary and orders.

Table 6.1 shows the essential information that a hospitalist program must transmit when a patient is discharged from a hospitalist's care, depending on the follow-up facility.

| Table | 6.1 | Flow of information at patient discharge |

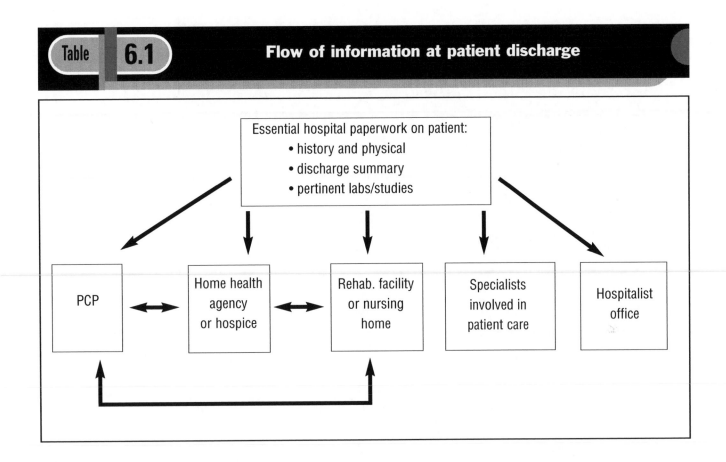

Flow of information at discharge

Communication at the time of a patient's discharge can be accomplished several ways. A telephone call that outlines essential information (such as medications, outstanding studies, and a follow-up plan) is likely the most efficient. However, other means (e.g., voicemail) are appropriate, especially if the discharge occurs after hours or on a weekend. Many hospitalist programs use a preprinted discharge form that can be faxed or communicated via e-mail. The information in this document should include the following (at a minimum):

- Discharge diagnoses
- A list of discharge medications
- Disposition
- Plans for communicating the results of any outstanding studies
- Required follow-up studies/appointments with timeline

Regardless of the mode of communication used, the discharge summary should be viewed and transmitted as a priority on the day of the patient's discharge. Information should be dictated in the following order:

1. Patient's name

2. Medical record number

3. Admission date

4. Discharge date

5. PCP's name

6. Admission diagnosis

7. Discharge diagnosis (final principal diagnosis)

8. Secondary discharge diagnosis

9. Consultations

10. Procedures

11. Brief summary of admission history and physical examination

12. Pertinent lab, x-ray and special studies

13. Summary of hospital course

14. Complications

15. Condition at discharge

16. Disposition

17. Discharge plan and physician follow-up

   • diet

   • activity level

   • ancillary services (home health, physical therapy, case management, etc.)

   • medication list at the time of admission

   • medication list at the time of discharge

   • required follow-up studies/appointments, including a timeline

18. Pending test results

19. DNR status

As noted, a telephone call from the hospitalist or hospitalist service to the patient within 48 hours of discharge reinforces the discharge plan.

Facilitating communication via electronic means

To ensure patient safety and continuity of care, hospitalists must not only establish strong communication links with PCPs, specialists, and patients but also with other hospitalists in the program, nurses, and other providers. For hospitalists programs that span multiple hospitals and numerous sites, this process becomes even more complex.

As a result, some hospitalist programs are turning to electronic means of communication (e.g., Web logs, patient "portals"—or sites that offer a broad array of resources and services, etc.) to keep all parties informed and up-to-date on patients' status.

Figure 6.1 shows one facility's reasoning and process for establishing communication pathways via a Web log accessible to physicians via the organization's Intranet.

Figure 6.2 shows one facility's plan for communication data between hospital and outpatient clinics in lieu of an electronic medical records system.

Communicating the admission protocol

It is good practice for a hospitalist program to clearly communicate to referring physicians, hospitalists, and other providers affiliated with the hospitalist program the protocol for admitting patients into the hospitalist service.

Figure 6.3 is the admissions protocol for one hospitalist program, including communication expectations for hospitalists and referring providers.

Surveying referring providers

Ideally, hospitalist programs systematically monitor all forms of communication to referring physicians to gain feedback about the effectiveness of the program. However, such an endeavor can be difficult and time/resource consuming. As a result, it may be more practical to gather periodic feedback from referring physicians in the form of physician satisfaction surveys. Remember, feedback can be garnered in less formal ways as well, such as through periodic phone calls.

Figures 6.4, 6.5, and 6.6 are sample forms for surveying the referring physicians who use your hospitalist service.

Surveying other providers

In addition to gathering periodic feedback from referring physicians, do not forget the other providers who may have special insight into how your program may be improved. These providers include physician assistants, nurses, and other support staff.

Figures 6.7 and 6.8 are surveys of nurse satisfaction with the hospitalist program. Both can be easily tailored to survey any provider who works with the hospitalists on a daily basis.

Figure 6.1   **Establishing communication pathways via a Web log**

Why implement a Web log?

An effective tool was needed for communication between

- the hospitalists and the hospital's 10 outpatient clinics
- hospitalists across the various shifts
- the hospitalists and nursing staff

The clerical staff members in the hospitalist service see patients within 24 hours of admission. They confirm the identity of each patient's primary care physician (PCP), advise patients about how to contact the hospitalist service, and let them know which hospitalist will care for them during their hospital stays. Patients' data (e.g., PCP, hospitalist, and some basic admission information) is entered into an Intranet-based Web log. This log contains both inpatients and discharged patients, and is archived for six months. The PCP is informed via e-mail or a phone call when a patient has been admitted.

Each clinic physician can view these logs at any time to see if they have patients who are hospitalized. Hospitalists use a different log to communicate patient information regarding admissions and cross-coverage issues to the physician who resumes care within the hospitalist service. The Web log contains the names of the physicians making rounds each day, as well as their pager numbers, so that the nursing staff knows which hospitalist to contact daily for each patient, and print on demand.

Implementation plan:

When a patient is discharged from the hospitalist service, the patient's PCP is notified, and he or she can access the patient's discharge summary on the Web log to view

- patient demographic information
- a brief summary of why the patient was admitted
- the patient's discharge date, disposition, and any follow-up appointments

This information enables all physicians affiliated with the hospitalist program access to patients' data (i.e., the Web log serves as our "chart"), in the absence of an electronic medical record for our hospital.

The information about patient admission and discharges contained in the Web log is also communicated to the hospital's outpatient clinics via e-mail. Staff at the outpatient sites have "read only" access to the Web log to view and print patient information needed for when the patient returns to the outpatient office for a follow-up. All patient information entered into the Web log, as well as physician schedules, are updated by the clerical staff and maintained daily. This information is considered a communication tool and not part of the patient's record.

*Source: **Mary Dallas, MD and Revathi A-Davidson, MPH**, Presbyterian Healthcare Services/Presbyterian Hospital, Albuquerque, NM. Albuquerque, NM.*

Figure 6.2 — Communication between hospital and outpatient clinics in lieu of an electronic medical records system

Why implement electronic communication to outpatient clinics?

Robert Wachter, MD, professor of medicine at the University of California, San Francisco, has referred to the "voltage drop," or the loss of information across the hospital threshold. The Web log (see **Figure 6.1**) represents a communication pathway we have created to ensure that the voltage drop is kept to a minimum. In addition, absent an electronic solution and at the request of the hospitalists, we have begun a new process that involves communicating basic patient care information from the PCP at the time of admission.

Because Presbyterian Healthcare Services does not yet have an enterprise-wide electronic medical record system, obtaining relevant clinical information at the time of admission has been difficult. The hospitalists identified the following four items they would like to gather when a Presbyterian clinic patient is admitted:

- Patient's medication list
- Patient's problem list
- Patient's last clinic note
- Any advance directives

Implementation plan:

Once the clinic is notified of an admission, the above four clinical items are obtained from the patient's clinic record by the clinic's medical records department and faxed to the hospitalist office. This was begun as a pilot with just one of the larger Presbyterian clinics. However, given the positive feedback from the hospitalists about how useful it is to have this information, the system will be rolled out to the remaining nine clinics.

*Source: **Mary Dallas, MD,** and **Revathi A-Davidson, MPH,** Presbyterian Healthcare Services/Presbyterian Hospital, Albuquerque, NM.*

Figure **6.3** — Admission protocol, including communication expectations for hospitalists and referring providers

I. Patient selection

- Patients over 15 years of age with an acute or chronic medical illness who cannot adequately be cared for in an outpatient setting.
- Patients over 15 years of age with an acute medical or surgical illness who may (but do not definitely) require surgery.
- Patients over 15 years of age who require surgery but who have a comorbid medical condition requiring ongoing medical care.

II. Process

- Referring physician will call the admitting physician on hospitalist service to relay the reasons for admission and to receive acceptance for medical evaluation.
- Referring physician will supply the medical record with the patient or will fax relevant information from the medical record to the admitting physician.
- Transfer information: Information to be supplied to the hospitalist at the time of admission should include the following:

  -Brief history of present illness

  -Past medical and surgical history, including co-morbid conditions

  -Current medications

  -Medication allergies

  -Legal next of kin

  -Do not resuscitate status/living will status

  -Discharge/transfer summary when appropriate

III. Admission discrepancy/borderline admissions

When there is a difference of opinion about the admission of a patient to the hospital, the hospitalist is expected to provide a reason why admission is not warranted, as well as an alternative outpatient management plan.

Figure 6.3   **Admission protocol, including communication expectations for hospitalists and referring providers (cont.)**

IV. Admission to *(name of hospitalist service/hospital)*

- Admitting physician will supply a copy of the admitting history, physical examination, and plan of care to the referring physician within one hour of evaluation.
- *(Name of hospitalist service)* will provide updates with significant changes in clinical status and at discharge.
- *(Name of hospitalist service)* will involve the referring physician in any major diagnostic treatment plans.
- *(Name of hospitalist service)* will work with the referring physician to plan the discharge of patient.
- *(Name of hospitalist service)* will supply a dictated discharge summary within three hours of discharge

Source: Written by **Kenneth G. Simone, DO,** *founder and president, Hospitalist and Practice Solutions, Veazie, ME, for Northeast Inpatient Medical Services, St. Joseph Hospital, Bangor, ME.*

Figure	6.4	Referring physician satisfaction survey—Format 1

Your satisfaction with the hospitalist services provided at *(name of hospital)* is important to us. To help us serve you better in the future, please check the box that best describes how you feel about our services.

1. Are you satisfied with the quality of medical care delivered to your patients at *(name of hospital)*?

Yes [ ]   No [ ]

If not, please explain: _____.

2. Do you routinely distribute the *(name of hospital)* inpatient service brochure to your patients?

Yes [ ]   No [ ]

If not, please explain: _____.

3. When called upon, are you willing to assist *(name of hospitalist service)* in the management of your difficult hospitalized patient?   Yes [ ]   No [ ]

If not, please explain: _____.

4. Do your patients seem satisfied with the overall care delivered by *(name of hospitalist service)* during their hospital stays?   Yes [ ]   No [ ]

If not, please explain: _____.

5. Your overall satisfaction with *(name of hospitalist service)* is:

[ ] 1. Excellent   [ ] 2. Very good   [ ] 3. Good   [ ] 4. Fair   [ ] 5. Poor

Please provide any suggestions for improvement below:

_____

_____

_____

Source: Northeast Inpatient Medical Services, St. Joseph Hospital, Bangor, ME.

Figure 6.5 — **Referring physician satisfaction survey—Format 2**

Instructions:

For each statement below, please indicate the extent of your agreement or disagreement by placing a check in the appropriate box.

1. Did the communication between the hospitalist and you support continuity of care for your patient?

Not applicable	Strongly disagree	Neutral	Agree	Strongly agree

2. How soon after the patient's discharge did you receive the discharge summary?

Not applicable	Not received	More than 3 days	1–3 days	Within 24 hours

3. Overall, how satisfied are you with the hospitalist who provided care for your patient?

Not applicable	Very dissatisfied	Dissatisfied	Somewhat dissatisfied	Satisfied	Very satisfied

4. Overall, how satisfied are you with our hospitalist program?

Not applicable	Very dissatisfied	Dissatisfied	Somewhat dissatisfied	Satisfied	Very satisfied

5. In your opinion, are your patients satisfied with the care provided by our hospitalist program?

Not applicable	Very dissatisfied	Dissatisfied	Somewhat dissatisfied	Satisfied	Very satisfied

Figure 6.5 **Referring physician satisfaction survey—Format 2 (cont.)**

6. Practice location of physician completing this survey:
[City, state]

Please provide comments you may have regarding the *(name of hospitalist program)* **as a whole or any individual hospitalist with whom you have worked.**

Physician name:_____
Office phone:_____
E-mail:_____

Source: **Brian J. Bossard, MD,** *founder an director, Inpatient Physician Associates, Lincoln, NE.*

Figure 6.6   Referring physician satisfaction survey—Format 3

Your satisfaction with the hospitalist services provided at *(name of hospital)* is important to us. To help us serve you better in the future, please check the box that best describes how you feel about our services.

PATIENT INFORMATION (to be completed by *(name of hospital)* hospitalist or designated staff member)

Patient name_____   Admission date: _____

Primary care provider_____   Discharge date:_____

1. Admitted from: [ ] Doctors office   [ ] Emergency room   [ ] Direct from home   [ ] Nursing facility
[ ] Other

2. Admitted to: [ ] *(name of hospital)*   [ ] *(name of alternate facility, if applicable)*

INFORMATION FLOW (to be completed by patient's primary care physician)

3. I was informed of the patient's admission to *(name of hospital)*.   [ ]Yes   [ ] No

4. I received a copy of the patient's history and physical examination.   [ ]Yes   [ ] No

5. I received the patient's discharge summary in a timely manner.   [ ]Yes   [ ] No

6. I was informed of the patient's progress on a regular basis.   [ ]Yes   [ ] No

COMMUNICATION (to be completed by patient's primary care physician)

7. Grade the *(name of hospitalist program)* hospitalists in terms of how well they involved you in your patient's treatment plan:
[ ] Excellent   [ ]Very good   [ ]Good   [ ]Fair   [ ] Poor

8. Were you in agreement with the treatment plan?   [ ]Yes   [ ] No
If not, please explain: _____.

Figure 6.6   **Referring physician satisfaction survey—Format 3 (cont.)**

9. Was the discharge plan appropriate?   [ ] Yes   [ ] No
If not, please explain: _____.

10. Was the discharge summary complete?   [ ] Yes   [ ] No
If not, please explain: _____.

11. My patients' opinion the overall care he or she received at *(name of hospital)* was:
   [ ] Excellent   [ ] Very good   [ ] Good   [ ] Fair   [ ] Poor

12. My overall satisfaction with the hospitalist services at *(name of hospital)* is:
   [ ] Excellent   [ ] Very good   [ ] Good   [ ] Fair   [ ] Poor

Source: Northeast Inpatient Medical Services, St. Joseph Hospital, Bangor, ME.

Figure 6.7 — **Nurse satisfaction survey—Format 1**

Instructions:

For each statement below, please indicate the extent of your agreement or disagreement by placing a check in the appropriate box.

1. (Teamwork) The hospitalist physicians and nurses have a collaborative working relationship at _____ hospital.

Not applicable	Not sure	Strongly disagree	Disagree	Agree	Strongly agree

2. (Value) The hospitalist physicians value and respect nurses' input and collaboration as integral members of the healthcare team.

Not applicable	Not sure	Strongly disagree	Disagree	Agree	Strongly agree

3. (Teamwork) The hospitalist physicians and nurses communicate respectfully with each other.

Not applicable	Not sure	Strongly disagree	Disagree	Agree	Strongly agree

4. (Leadership) The hospitalist physicians and other physicians on the medical staff communicate directly with each other as appropriate without putting nurses in the middle.

Not applicable	Not sure	Strongly disagree	Disagree	Agree	Strongly agree

5. (Integrity) I feel comfortable calling the hospitalist physicians to clarify or obtain orders.

Not applicable	Not sure	Strongly disagree	Disagree	Agree	Strongly agree

6. (Teamwork) The hospitalist physicians take opportunities to teach staff.

Not applicable	Not sure	Strongly disagree	Disagree	Agree	Strongly agree

*Source: **Brian J. Bossard, MD,** founder and director, Inpatient Physician Associates, Lincoln, NE.*

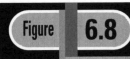

Nurse satisfaction survey—Format 2

Instructions:

Please answer each question by placing a check in the appropriate box. Return in the envelope provided by (date) to the (medical staff office, etc.).

Category	Question	Strongly agree (4)	Agree (3)	Disagree (2)	Strongly disagree (1)	Not sure (0)
Teamwork	The hospitalist physicians and nurses have a collaborative working relationship at *(name of hospital)*.					
Value	The hospitalist physicians value and respect nurses' input and collaboration as integral members of the healthcare team.					
Teamwork	The hospitalist physicians and nurses communicate respectfully with each other.					
Leadership	The hospitalist physicians and other physicians on the medical staff communicate directly with each other as appropriate without putting nurses in the middle.					
Integrity	I feel comfortable calling the hospitalist physicians to clarify or obtain orders.					
Teamwork	The hospitalist physicians take opportunities to teach staff.					

Figure	6.8	Nurse satisfaction survey—Format 2 (cont.)

Check one: [ ] Registered nurse   [ ] Licensed practical nurse

Name (optional):_____

Suggestions regarding the *(name of hospital)* hospitalist program:

_____

_____

_____

Comments regarding individual hospitalists:

_____

_____

_____

*Source: **Brian J. Bossard, MD**, founder and director, Inpatient Physician Associates, Lincoln, NE.*

Communication
with patients

7

Communication with patients

Diane Craig, MD, FACP

Patient satisfaction is good medicine for patients, physicians, and hospitals. Studies show that satisfied patients may recover faster and better, are less likely to sue, and can give hospitals a competitive advantage.

Consider, too, that patient satisfaction is poised to become even more important. Starting in 2006, hospitals across the country will begin using the Hospital-Consumer Assessment of Health Care Providers and Systems (H-CAHPS, *www.cahps.ahrq.gov/default.asp*) to survey and voluntarily report patient satisfaction data to the Centers for Medicare & Medicaid Services (CMS). CMS plans to initiate public reporting of those results in late 2007. This information will enable patients—who are well on their way to becoming savvy medical consumers—to compare hospitals in their communities.

In a practice known as "pay for performance" some institutions have even begun to link patient satisfaction scores to physicians' compensation. The reason? There is a growing movement toward ensuring that physicians maintain a personal investment in their patients' satisfaction.

With the above in mind, directors of hospital medicine programs and hospitalists should strive to understand what factors lead to high levels of satisfaction among hospitalized patients and what interventions have proven to be successful in improving patients' experiences.

Because of the efforts by CMS to develop a consistent, nationwide tool, learning more about the H-CAHPS tool and the process for its implementation would be a reasonable place to start. In addition, the Society of Hospital Medicine (SHM, *www.hospitalmedicine.org*) also provides guidance on developing and administering patient satisfaction surveys.

Measure patient satisfaction

To provide physicians with critical patient satisfaction information, hospitalist programs should identify, measure, and collect the data that will be most useful. Although many hospitals turn to third-party organizations, such as Press Ganey (*www.pressganey.com*) or NRC+Picker (www.*nrcpicker.com*), to help them develop systems for capturing patient satisfaction information, you can also design your own survey process.

Before getting additional diagnostic information, consider how that information will change your management. Ask questions that will allow you to understand and act on the feedback. Notably, the H-CAHPS survey will include questions in the following six domains:

- Nurse-to-patient communication
- Nursing services
- Physician-to-patient communication
- Physical environment
- Pain control
- Communication to patients about medications

The following are possible questions to include in your own survey that specifically focus on physician-to-patient communication:

- Did the hospitalist spend adequate time with you?
- Did the hospitalist display adequate concern for your condition/treatment?
- Was there sufficient time to ask the hospitalist questions and relay any worries?
- Did the hospitalist keep you informed throughout your hospital stay?
- Was the hospitalist courteous and considerate?
- Were you satisfied with the hospitalist's manner of communication?
- Was the hospitalist available to meet with family members?

Keep patient satisfaction out in the open

Finally, remember that feedback from patients regarding their hospital experience should be out in the open. The indicators your facility chooses for measuring patient satisfaction should be shared widely with all members of the healthcare team, including hospitalists. When hospitalists know which skills are being specifically measured, they will likely focus even more attention on them, which can only improve the overall impression patients have of their hospital stays.

Figures 7.1, and 7.2, and are forms for surveying patients who have recently been under the care of a hospitalist in your program.

Marketing outreach for starting and expanding a hospitalist program

Although inpatient medicine is entering its second decade, many patients and their families have not yet been exposed to hospitalists. In addition, the popularity and growth of hospital medicine has led most primary care physicians to realize the advantages of the inpatient model of care, but many still harbor misconceptions about "losing" patients to hospitalists, or simply do not have all the facts about what a partnership with a hospitalist program entails. For these reasons, marketing outreach to the community is vital to the success of an inpatient medicine program.

Education of and communication with the medical community can be accomplished in a variety of ways. Drafting a detailed letter describing hospitalist practice and services is certainly a starting point. Additionally, a hospitalist brochure sent to referring providers' offices for distribution to patients could reinforce the practice's objectives and educate the patients in the community. The hospitalist program's clinical director or another representative of the service should follow up on these initiatives with a visit to the offices of referring providers. At these meetings, the program's objectives, mission, services offered, and expectations can be discussed in detail. In addition, the representative can distribute to referring physicians a practice manual containing

- relevant program policies
- procedures offered
- program expectations (from both the referring physician's and hospitalist's perspective)
- hospitalists' short biographies, with photos

Figure 7.1   Patient satisfaction survey—Format 1

To be completed by the recent patient of *(name of hospital/hospitalist service)*

Instructions:

For each statement below, please indicate the extent of your agreement or disagreement by placing a check in the appropriate box.

1. **How would you rate the daily visits made by your hospital physician (time spent, quality of visit)?**

Excellent	Very good	Good	Fair	Poor

2. **How would you rate your hospitalist's ability to communicate with you (listening, giving clear explanations)?**

Excellent	Very good	Good	Fair	Poor

3. **How would you rate your hospitalist's ability to communicate with your family (listening, giving clear explanations)?**

Excellent	Very good	Good	Fair	Poor

4. **How would you rate the way you were treated by the hospitalist (kindness, respect, dignity)?**

Excellent	Very good	Good	Fair	Poor

5. **How would you rate the overall medical care that you received from the hospitalist?**

Excellent	Very good	Good	Fair	Poor

6. **Who was your hospitalist?**

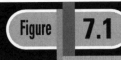

Patient satisfaction survey—Format 1 (cont.)

7. Was a physician assistant or nurse practitioner involved in your care?

8. If yes, can you identify him/her?

Please provide any additional comments you may have regarding the [name of hospital] hospitalist program as a whole, or any individual hospitalist who treated you.

FOR OFFICE USE ONLY

Patient's admission date:

Patient was admitted from: [ ] Doctor's office   [ ] Emergency room
[ ] Direct from home   [ ] Nursing facility   [ ] Other

Discharged to:

Primary Care Physician:
Physician name:_____
Office phone:_____
Email:_____

Source: Northeast Inpatient Medical Services, St. Joseph Hospital, Bangor, ME.

Figure 7.2 — Patient satisfaction survey—Format 2

To be completed by recent patient of *(name of hospital/hospitalist service)*

Instructions:
For each statement below, please indicate the extent of your agreement or disagreement by placing a check in the appropriate box.

1. Were you satisfied with the quality of medical care delivered in the hospital?

Not applicable	Very dissatisfied	Dissatisfied	Somewhat dissatisfied	Satisfied	Very satisfied

2. Were you satisfied with the quality of medical care received from the hospitalist who cared for you?

Not applicable	Very dissatisfied	Dissatisfied	Somewhat dissatisfied	Satisfied	Very satisfied

3. Did you feel that your medical care was coordinated well among the physicians caring for you?

Not applicable	Very dissatisfied	Dissatisfied	Somewhat dissatisfied	Satisfied	Very satisfied

4. Did the hospitalist treat you with respect, kindness, and dignity?

Not applicable	Very dissatisfied	Dissatisfied	Somewhat dissatisfied	Satisfied	Very satisfied

5. Did your hospitalist spend adequate time with you and your family explaining your condition?

Not applicable	Very dissatisfied	Dissatisfied	Somewhat dissatisfied	Satisfied	Very satisfied

6. Did your hospitalist conduct himself/herself in a professional manner?

Not applicable	Very dissatisfied	Dissatisfied	Somewhat dissatisfied	Satisfied	Very satisfied

7. Were you seen by a hospitalist each day?

Yes	No

© 2006 HCPro, Inc.
TOOLS AND STRATEGIES FOR AN EFFECTIVE HOSPITALIST PROGRAM

Figure 7.2 — Patient satisfaction survey—Format 2 (cont.)

8. Were you satisfied with your discharge plan?

Not applicable	Very dissatisfied	Dissatisfied	Somewhat dissatisfied	Satisfied	Very satisfied

9. Rate your overall satisfaction with [name of hospitalist service]:

Excellent	Very good	Good	Fair	Poor

10. Rate your overall satisfaction with the hospitalist who cared for you:

Excellent	Very good	Good	Fair	Poor

Please provide any additional comments you may have regarding the *[name of hospital]* hospitalist program as a whole, or any individual hospitalist who cared for you.

FOR OFFICE USE ONLY

Patient's admission date:

Patient was admitted from: [ ] Doctor's office   [ ] Emergency room
[ ] Direct from home   [ ] Nursing facility   [ ] Other

Discharged to:

Primary Care Physician:
Physician name:_____
Office phone:_____
E-mail:_____

Source: Northeast Inpatient Medical Services, St. Joseph Hospital, Bangor, ME.

Developing a practice Web site is another form of outreach to both the medical and lay community. The site can be formulated to communicate with the local and outlying communities (providers and patients) and may serve as a recruitment tool.

Figure 7.3 is one hospitalist program's draft communication plan for a hospitalist program launch. **Figure 7.4** is the corresponding letter to referring physicians in the community announcing the new inpatient medicine program.

Figure 7.5 is a draft communication plan for the expansion of a hospitalist program to a second hospital/medical center site. **Figure 7.6** is the corresponding letter to referring physicians in the community announcing the expansion plan.

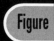

Figure 7.3 Draft communication plan for a hospitalist program launch

Overall messages

- Hospitalists will provide continuity of care for inpatients at *(name of hospital)*.
- Hospitalists will coordinate inpatient care for patients admitted through the emergency department (ED) who do not have a primary care physician (PCP); provide general care and consultative general care as requested from members of the medical staff; provide care for patients transferred to *(name of hospital)* from outside *(name of city)* as referred by the physician from outside *(name of city)*; respond to requests for patient evaluation as required by the restraint/seclusion policy; respond to code blue requests; respond to inpatient emergencies as requested by the attending physician; work with specialists as needed; and provide discharge planning for patients, which may include identifying a physician for the patient or providing information to the patient's referring physician.
- Hospitalists will help manage the patient-placement process and may help facilitate patient moves. This model ensures that patients will receive appropriate levels of care, intensive care/progressive care beds are free, and quality patient care is maintained. Hospitalists also will help facilitate timely patient discharges and arrangements for any posthospital care needed.
- Hospitalists will aid physicians who are busy in their offices by providing consults or by responding to emergencies situations for a physician's hospitalized patient.
- Hospitalists can accept patients from out-of-town physicians who do not know where to refer their patients.

Physician communication avenues

- Hold meetings with physician groups, including
    - ED physicians

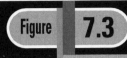

**Draft communication plan for
a hospitalist program launch (cont.)**

- Trauma team leaders

- Psychiatrists

- Other key physician groups

- Submit an article about the program to *(name of hospital)* publications

- Develop a letter and brochure for *(name of hospital)* medical staff and include the paperwork (forms) necessary for referrals

- Develop a separate mailing for referring physicians that promotes a phone number for making referrals to the hospitalist (possibly conduct the phone referral line through the nurse on-call program)

- Send a hospitalist program representative to attend a new-physician event at *(name of hospital)* to provide information about the program

Medical staff center
- Set up an informational meeting with all staff from key areas throughout the medical center who will be involved in making the program a success and who need to be aware of the program. Describe the program, introduce our new hospitalists, and answer questions. Offer meetings at two different times. Invite patient family representatives, as well key staff members or departmental representatives to relay information back to the staff. These may include

    - ED staff

    - house supervisors

    - medical records staff

    - discharge planners

    - mental health staff

    - nurse on-call staff

- Hold a hospitalist program reception event for medical center staff members.

Volunteers
- Include information about the program in *(name of hospital)* volunteer newsletter

Public
- Send a press release to news outlets about the start of the hospitalist program (working with the public relations department)

- Follow up with local media

*Source: **Brian J. Bossard, MD,** founder and director, Inpatient Physician Associates, Lincoln, NE.*

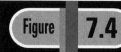

Letter to referring physicians announcing hospitalist program launch

(Date)

Dear Physician:

(Name of hospitalist service) began hospitalist services at *(name of hospital)* on *(date)*. Hospitalists are available 24 hours a day, seven days a week to provide adult inpatient care. In addition to myself, the five full-time internists associated with *(name of hospitalist service)* include Drs. *(physicians' names)*.

The enclosed brochure provides detailed information about our program and instructions on how to refer a patient to *(name of hospitalist service)*. We will provide care to hospitalized patients who do not have a physician and to hospitalized patients referred to us by other physicians for inpatient care or for consults.

An issue of interest to the medical staff is the primary care call coverage for the unassigned adult patient population. *(Name of hospitalist service)* physicians will assume responsibility for the care of these patients who require inpatient general medical care. At the time of discharge, these patients often require follow-up care with a local primary care physician. *(Name of hospitalist service)* will continue the current system for discharge management for unassigned patients. This system uses the primary care call rotation to arrange for posthospital follow-up care (as is the practice for patients discharged from the emergency department) and is especially important for unassigned patients with acute-care problems.

You may not feel comfortable providing outpatient follow-up care for a patient you have not cared for in the medical center. If you have an interest in participating in the inpatient care of the unassigned patient population, please do not hesitate to contact me. Unless I hear from you, we will follow this plan to care for unassigned patients.

Our mission is to provide comprehensive, efficient, and service-oriented inpatient medical care for your adult patients. Utilization of *(name of hospitalist service)* services is voluntary. The emergency department physicians will continue to contact you if you have a patient in the emergency department who requires admission. If you elect to have *(name of hospitalist service)* care for your patient during hospitalization, you simply need to inform the emergency department physician and he or she will contact our service. We also are available in-house to respond to consultations.

Figure 7.4

Letter to referring physicians announcing hospitalist program launch (cont.)

The physicians of *(name of hospitalist service)* are excited about getting started. Should you have any questions regarding the hospitalist program, please don't hesitate to contact me by phone at *(telephone number)* or via e-mail at *(e-mail address)*.

Sincerely,

(Name of hospitalist director), MD, FACP
Director, *(Name of hospitalist service)*

Source: **Brian J. Bossard, MD,** *founder and director, Inpatient Physician Associates, Lincoln, NE.*

Figure 7.5   Draft communication plan for a hospitalist program expansion

Overall messages:

- Hospitalist service expands to *(name of second facility)* beginning *(date).*

- Hospitalists will provide continuity of care for inpatients at both *(names of facilities).* This service is in keeping with our mission to improve standard of care and takes patient care to the next level by having a physician available in-house at all times.

- Medical center/health system benefits by having hospitalists at multiple sites:
    - Hospitalists help move patients to the most appropriate level of care (aids in freeing up beds)
    - Hospitalists are available to work with hospital staff (nurses, technicians) to better determine needs of patients
    - Referring physicians benefit by having to make fewer hospital visits, having a resource for consults, and being informed about patients' care
    - Patients benefit through faster discharge times and lower readmission rates; patients like having a physician available to talk with them and their family members at any time during their hospital stay

- Hospitalists are experienced physicians who provide safe, effective patient care. There will be an emphasis on teamwork between the hospitalist/referring physician and the hospitalist/medical center staff members, as well as a focus on using teamwork to improve patient care (i.e., improved efficiency, more standardized care for optimal outcomes).

- Hospitalists in the *(name of hospitalist service)* will do the following:

    - Coordinate inpatient care for patients who are admitted through the emergency department and who do not have a primary care physician
    - Provide general medical care and consultative general care as requested by members of the medical staff
    - Provide care for patients who are referred by an out-of-town physician
    - Respond to requests for patient evaluation as required by the restraint/seclusion policy
    - Respond to rapid response/Code blue requests
    - Respond to inpatient emergencies as requested by attending physician

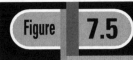

Figure 7.5 | Draft communication plan for a hospitalist program expansion (cont.)

- Work with specialists as needed
- Provide discharge planning for patients, which may include identifying a physician for the patient or providing information to the patient's referring physician

- Hospitalists help manage the patient placement process and may help facilitate patient moves to appropriate levels of care, which will free up intensive care/progressive care beds while maintaining the quality of patient care.

- Hospitalists also help facilitate timely discharges and arrangements for any posthospital care needed.

- Hospitalists can help physicians who are busy with patients in their offices by providing consults or by responding to emergency situations for a physician's hospitalized patient and providing follow-up to the physician.

- Hospitalists can accept patients from out-of-town physicians who do not know where to refer their patients; hospitalists can provide care and arrange for other physicians who need to be involved in the care.

Source: **Brian J. Bossard, MD,** *founder and director, Inpatient Physician Associates, Lincoln, NE.*

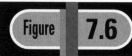

Letter to referring physicians announcing hospitalist program expansion

---

(Date)

Dear Physician:

(Name of hospitalist service) will expand hospitalist services to *(name of hospital)* on *(date)*. *(Name of hospitalist service)* hospitalists are available 24 hours a day, seven days a week to provide adult inpatient care.

I am pleased to announce five new full-time internists associated with *(name of hospitalist service)*: Drs. *(names of physicians)*.

The enclosed brochure provides detailed information on our program and instructions on how to refer a patient to the hospitalist service. We will provide care to adult hospitalized patients who do not have a primary care physician and adult hospitalized patients referred to us by other physicians for inpatient care or for consults.

Our mission is to provide comprehensive, efficient, and service-oriented inpatient medical care for your adult patients. Use of *(name of hospitalist service)* services is voluntary. The emergency department (ED) physicians will continue to contact you if you have a patient in the ED who requires admission. If you elect to have *(name of hospitalist service)* care for your patient during hospitalization, you simply need to inform the ED physician and he or she will contact our service. We also are available in-house to respond to consultations.

We are excited about providing care for your patients at both *(name of hospital)* sites. Should you have any questions regarding the hospitalist program, please don't hesitate to contact me by phone, *(phone number),* or via e-mail, *(e-mail address).*

Sincerely,

(Name of hospitalist program director) MD, FACP
Director, *(Name of hospitalist service)*

Source: **Brian J. Bossard, MD,** *founder and director, inpatient physician Associates, Lincoln, NE.*

Develop a brochure to inform patients about the hospitalist service

Why create a brochure? Hospitalist medicine is still in its infancy, and most patients are being placed under the care of a hospitalist for the first time. They may not understand why their PCPs are not their attending physicians. A patient-oriented brochure can help explain the new system. In addition, business cards created for each of the hospitalists in the service provide patients and their families with easily accessible contact information.

Elements of a hospitalist brochure

A comprehensive hospitalist program brochure addresses, at a minimum, the following basic patient questions:

- What is a hospitalist?
- What is the relationship between the hospitalist and my PCP?
- How does the hospitalist service work?
- What if I need another specialist while I'm in the hospital?
- How can the hospitalist service/individual hospitalists be contacted?
- What can I expect during my hospitalization?
- Will my PCP be kept up to date about my progress during my hospitalist stay?

If it is general practice to have a hospitalist service staff member visit each patient within 24 hours of admission, he or she may hand out the brochure at that time, pointing out which hospitalist will care for the patient. When the hospitalist meets the patient, he or she can leave a business card for the patient and his or her family. Alternatively, the hospitalist may present the brochure upon introduction to each patient, describing how the service works and answering any initial questions.

Hospitalist service brochures are also frequently given to outpatient clinics so that information about the service can be shared upstream of an inpatient episode.

Note: To view a sample hospitalist program brochure that does not appear in the book, refer to the CD-ROM that accompanies this book.

Hospitalist performance reviews

8

Hospitalist performance reviews

Kenneth G. Simone, DO

Jeffrey R. Dichter, MD, FACP

Changing culture

In medicine, possibly more than in any other profession, a substandard performance may lead to loss of life, and it can have legal implications for the healthcare provider. As a result, the medical profession and federal healthcare regulators, among others, are grappling with questions such as the following:

- How does one measure physician competency?
- What is quality, and how is it measured?
- How could the medical system guarantee its "customers" that all providers are competent?
- What regulations appropriately evaluate and ensure patient safety?
- How are providers who have exhibited substandard performance dealt with?

In the 21st century, the healthcare industry is evaluating and changing the culture in which it has operated for hundreds of years. It is moving away from anecdotal care toward implementing evidenced-based medicine, improving patient safety, and promoting quality initiatives. Essentially, the healthcare industry is attempting to standardize medical care. It is addressing the unnecessary errors and deaths in hospitals caused either by an ineffective or faulty system or by poor patient care.

The healthcare industry is looking "outside the box," turning to and learning from non-medical industries (e.g., aviation) in search of safety and quality assurance systems. For this initiative to be successful, the healthcare industry realizes that it must restructure a system in which providers are afraid of admitting their mistakes (and of asking for help) for fear of harsh penalties and possible loss of their medical licenses and careers.

In the meantime, those involved in the evaluation and assurance of quality care and competency are responsible for providing clear and concise feedback to each provider and identifying areas of needed improvement. When appropriate, educational forums may be offered.

In addition, considering the high degree of scrutiny on physicians' performance by the Joint Commission on Accreditation of Healthcare Organizations (JCAHO) and the Centers for Medicare & Medicaid Services (CMS), state medical boards, and hospitals' own quality mechanisms, evaluating hospitalists' job performance should be a high priority for inpatient medicine programs.

However, there is more to performance reviews than ensuring that your hospitalists make the grade with regard to safety, quality, and patient satisfaction. The most successful programs care about, monitor, and provide feedback to hospitalists in an effort to improve their performance and facilitate professional growth. Specifically, the performance review process provides hospitalists with the opportunity to set personal goals that improve the overall hospitalist service.

Although the standards found in the "Medical Staff" and "Performance Improvement" chapters of the JCAHO's *Comprehensive Accreditation Manual for Hospitals* require hospitals to evaluate physician performance at reappointment (**MS.4.40**) and analyze aggregate performance improvement data (**PI.2.10**) on an ongoing basis, the Joint Commission does not mandate specific content for physician performance reviews.

Evaluation should not just involve reviewing the hospitalists at reappointment (see section below on "Added benefits of conducting regular reviews") but rather should be done annually by the hospitalist practice itself.

Roadblocks to evaluating performance

The successful design and implementation of a performance feedback system requires time, energy, and medical staff resources. All of these elements are in short supply within busy inpatient medicine programs. Is it worth the effort to conduct individual performance reviews—and do the reviews actually result in better performance and improved patient care? The short answer is yes.

Physician managers often find performance reviews a difficult task for various reasons:

- The practice of evaluating what makes a "good" hospitalist does not easily lend itself to analysis

- Observations of hospitalists' daily rounds can be time consuming and/or impractical for busy hospitalist programs

- Autonomy has long been a main tenet of the medical profession, and physicians are reluctant to judge other physicians' work styles

- Peer or subordinate performance review is not typically taught in medical school, and there is a dearth of external resources to aid physician managers in this task

- Most hospitalists' job descriptions are not comprehensive enough to serve as the foundation for measuring their performance

Clearly delineate expectations

Physicians are achievers by nature, selection, and training. Therefore, if you tell hospitalists precisely what is expected of them in virtually any aspect of their performance, the vast majority will meet and usually exceed those expectations.

It is imperative to let hospitalists know the following:

- At what intervals they can expect to be evaluated (e.g., 60 days post-hire, six months post-hire, and annually thereafter)
- On what criteria they will be evaluated

- Who will conduct their evaluations (both the data-gathering phase and the actual review)
- What "tools" will be used to measure their performance (e.g., patient satisfaction surveys, length of stay numbers, readmissions, etc.)
- What opportunities they will have to give feedback on the results of the evaluation

Consider drafting a brief outline discussing these points and distributing it to both new hospitalists and those already on staff. The evaluation should, at a minimum, include the expectations of the provider as communicated through the job description. Take care to protect the evaluation process findings from any individual except those on a "need to know" basis. Doing so will foster an honest and frank discussion and a corrective plan for any of the provider's shortcomings and errors and serve as an educational rather than a punitive tool.

Figure 8.1 shows one hospitalist program's departmental guidelines for conducting hospitalists' performance evaluations.

Added benefits of conducting regular reviews

Hospitalist performance reviews, when done successfully, can provide guidance during the physician reappointment process, an important hospital function. At bare minimum, all JCAHO-accredited organizations should review hospitalists' performance periodically to provide meaningful data at the time of their reappointment.

Figures 8.2 and **8.3** are sample forms for evaluating hospitalists' job performance.

Figure 8.4 is a sample form for evaluating the job performance of physician assistants who work within a hospitalist program.

Figure 8.1 — **Departmental guidelines for evaluating hospitalists' performance**

Each hospitalist will be evaluated at three months post-hire, at one year post-hire, and annually thereafter unless otherwise specified. The evaluation will cover (but is not limited to) the provider's

1. clinical performance
2. teamwork
3. appropriate communication and voicemail use
4. timely submission of patient billing information
5. physician satisfaction survey
6. patient satisfaction survey
7. coding and revenue reviews
8. adherence to the policy/procedure manual
9. adherence to medical staff requirements
10. attendance at required meetings

In addition, the evaluation will include input from the clinical director and administrative director at *(name of hospital)*. All contract negotiations will be coordinated through the chief executive officer and administrative director at *(name of hospital)*.

All admissions will take place at *(name of hospital)* unless the service cannot be provided at this institution.

*Source: Written by **Kenneth G. Simone, DO,** founder and president, Hospitalist and Practice Solutions, Veazie, ME, for Northeast Inpatient Medical Services, St. Joseph Hospital, Bangor, ME.*

Figure	8.2	Hospitalist performance evaluation—Format 1

Name: Date:

Position: Hospitalist   Anniversary Date:

Division: Date of hire:

5	EXCELLENT	Distinguished performance. Employee consistently and significantly exceeds performance standards.
4	CONSISTENTLY EXCEEDS STANDARDS	Above average performance. Employee consistently achieves and frequently exceeds performance standards.
3	CONSISTENTLY MEETS STANDARDS	Acceptable performance. Employee generally achieves performance standards and maintains a satisfactory performance level in most circumstances.
2	NEEDS IMPROVEMENT	Below average performance. Employee frequently does not achieve a satisfactory performance standard. Improvement is necessary.
1	UNSATISFACTORY	Unacceptable performance. Employee consistently fails to achieve performance standards. Substantial improvement is needed.
NA	NOT APPLICABLE	This rating does not apply to this position.

SECTION I: POSITION-SPECIFIC CRITERIA

Please check the box that most accurately describes the employee's performance over the entire period of evaluation.

Criteria:	1	2	3	4	5	N/A
Admits patients referred to the hospitalist service.						
Manages patient care during hospitalization.						
Develops treatment plans/directs treatment/performs credentialed procedures.						
Establishes a direct line of communication with the primary care physician when appropriate.						
Provides daily voicemail to referring providers as appropriate.						

| Figure | 8.2 | Hospitalist performance evaluation—Format 1 (cont.) |

	1	2	3	4	5	N/A
Develops a discharge plan and ensures that it is carried out.						
Submits patient charges daily.						
Strictly adheres to the *(name of hospitalist service)* policies and procedures.						
Works in a professional manner with nursing staff and other departments in patient-related matters.						
Carries out responsibilities as the supervising physician for mid-level providers.						
Prepares medical records on a timely basis per hospital requirements.						
Attends all required meetings.						
Meets all medical staff requirements.						
Teaches medical students/residents who may rotate through the medical service.						
Works with referring physicians to optimize the appropriate use of the integrated delivery system service.						
Develops *(name of hospitalist service)* clinical pathways, as appropriate: Work is performed at *(name of hospital)*.						
Maintains patient confidentiality.						

Comments:

_____

_____

_____

SECTION II: BEHAVIORAL CRITERIA

	1	2	3	4	5
Time management: Employee demonstrates an ability to prioritize work and complete essential tasks in a timely manner. Employee can perform multiple tasks, when necessary, without sacrificing accuracy.					
Judgment: Employee assesses situations from multiple perspectives and appropriately refers concerns to his or her supervisor. Employee uses the appropriate chain of command and makes good decisions under pressure.					

Figure **8.2**   Hospitalist performance evaluation—Format 1 (cont.)

	1	2	3	4	5
Supports mission: Employee supports the mission of *(name of hospitalist service)* and acts as a positive role model for other employees.					
Adapts to change: Employee adapts to change by willingly learning new policies and procedures. Employee offers constructive suggestions to help improve inpatient service's systems/processes.					
Attitude: Employee displays a positive attitude that reflects a belief in teamwork and the importance of supportive working relationships. Employee treats colleagues, patients, and visitors respectfully.					
Dependability: Employee shows dependability through attendance and punctuality. Employee shows an understanding of the needs of the division when scheduling time off.					
Customer service: Employee practices and promotes a high level of service to internal and external customers through timely, accurate, and courteous work. Anticipates the needs of internal and external customers, where appropriate.					
Accepts constructive criticism: Employee demonstrates the willingness to listen to and respond to constructive criticism through positive behavior changes. Does not exhibit defensive behavior during a discussion of problem areas.					

Comments:

_____

_____

_____

SECTION III: **PROGRESS TOWARD GOALS**

In the section below, please describe the progress made toward any goals set at a *previous* introductory or annual evaluation. Briefly describe goals:

Goal 1: [E.g., Jan. 2004—Set up system for code management]

 © 2006 HCPRO, INC.   TOOLS AND STRATEGIES FOR AN EFFECTIVE HOSPITALIST PROGRAM

Figure 8.2 Hospitalist performance evaluation—Format 1 (cont.)

❑ Exceeded expectations for performance

❑ Met expectations

❑ Continues to need improvement

Goal 2:

❑ Exceeded expectations for performance

❑ Met expectations

❑ Continues to need improvement

Comments:

_____

_____

_____

SECTION IV: SETTING NEW GOALS

Please identify two or three specific goals for the employee's development in the coming year. Progress toward these goals should be reviewed periodically during the year and at the next annual evaluation meeting. Employees should take an active role in setting goals for their own professional growth and development.

1. _____

_____

_____

_____

Figure	8.2	Hospitalist performance evaluation—Format 1 (cont.)

2. _____

_____

_____

_____

3. _____

_____

_____

_____

Additional Comments:

Employee Acknowledgment: My signature verifies that I have seen this evaluation but does not necessarily mean that I agree with my supervisor's assessment of my performance. I understand that I can attach comments to this evaluation if I choose and have those comments become part of my official personnel file in Human Resources.

Employee: _____   **Date:** _____

Supervisor: _____   **Date:** _____

Source: Northeast Inpatient Medical Services, St. Joseph Hospital, Bangor, ME.

Figure **8.3** **Hospitalist performance evaluation—Format 2**

Employee Name	Employment Date	Employee Department	Reviewing Manager
Date of Last Review	Current Review Date	Position Title	Date of Present Assignment

SECTION 1: DESCRIBE ASSIGNMENTS AND MAJOR RESPONSIBILITIES FOR THE REVIEW PERIOD (Add page if necessary)

Goal 1:
Goal 2:
Goal 3:
Etc.

SECTION 2: INDICATE WHETHER OR NOT GOALS WERE ACHIEVED

GOALS			COMPLETION COMMENTS
Goal 1	Achieved	Not Achieved	
Goal 2	Achieved	Not Achieved	
Goal 3	Achieved	Not Achieved	
Goal 4	Achieved	Not Achieved	
Goal 5	Achieved	Not Achieved	

SECTION 3: GENERAL COMMENTS AND SUMMARY RELATING TO THE STATUS AND ATTAINMENT OF THE ABOVE GOALS, THE DIFFICULTY OF THE GOALS, AND ANY FACTORS THAT COULD AFFECT THE ACHIEVMENT OF THE GOALS.

Figure 8.3   Hospitalist performance evaluation—Format 2 (cont.)

SECTION 4: EVALUATE AND DESCRIBE PERFORMANCE AND ACCOMPLISHMENTS USING THE FOLLOWING CRITERIA:

The following tables list suggested criteria for evaluating performance and are not intended to be all-inclusive. They may be changed, deleted, or added to as required. The comments area for each performance measure should be used for expansion, explanation, and description of the strengths and/or problem areas for each performance area. Enter "N/A" in those cases in which the performance area does not apply to this position.

Consistently, over time, performs all duties in an exceptional manner; significantly exceeds expectations with work of an exceptional quality, quantity, and timeliness; significantly exceeds all objectives and always achieves exceptional results well beyond those expected of the position. Note: highly limit your use of this rating.	EXCEPTIONAL 5
Consistently exceeds the normal expectations for the position; exceeds the criteria for the quality, quantity, and timeliness of work; consistently exceeds goals and objectives; achieves results beyond those expected for the position.	EXCEEDS 4
Consistently performs all duties of the position in a fully capable manner; meets all criteria for the quality, quantity, and timeliness of work; and meets goals and objectives.	MEETS 3
Performs many duties in a capable manner; meets some goals and objectives, but requires improvement in quality, quantity, and timeliness of work to achieve an overall satisfactory performance; may require more supervision than expected for assignment. Could be the performance level of those new to a position.	MARGINAL 2
Unacceptable performance that suggests a lack of willingness and/or ability to perform the requirements of the position. Separation or reassignment is indicated unless performance improves significantly. Requires excessive supervision.	UNSATISFACTORY 1

Figure	8.3	Hospitalist performance evaluation—Format 2 (cont.)

PERFORMANCE RESULTS

		Rating:
1.	**QUALITY OF WORK** Completes high-quality work with thoroughness and accuracy in achieving results. Thoroughly follows standards and procedures. Keeps complete records. Pays adequate attention to detail. Comments:	5 4 3 2 1
2.	**QUANTITY OF WORK** Completes assignments by or before deadline. Produces acceptable quantity of work. Maintains control of work regardless of environmental pressures. Manages priorities. Accepts new responsibilities. Comments:	5 4 3 2 1

PERFORMANCE FACTORS

		Rating:
3.	**JOB KNOWLEDGE AND TECHNICAL APPLICATION** Applies technical, professional knowledge to job requirements. Keeps job knowledge and technical skills current. Uses past experience to solve problems. Applies company and industry information. Comments:	5 4 3 2 1
4.	ORGANIZATION AND PLANNING Sets priorities, to optimize time usage. Engages in short- and long-term planning. Proposes milestones that allow progress to be adequately measured. Adheres to schedules and plans. Comments:	5 4 3 2 1
5.	ANALYTICAL AND PROBLEM SOLVING Understands and defines problems clearly. Formulates realistic solutions. Participates constructively in group problem solving. Anticipates and prevents problems. Comments:	5 4 3 2 1
6.	JUDGMENT AND DECISION MAKING Considers relevant alternatives before making decisions. Shows timeliness and	Rating:

Figure **8.3**   Hospitalist performance evaluation—Format 2 (cont.)

conviction in making recommendations and decisions that withstand critical examination. Comments:	5 4 3 2 1
7. SELF-IMPROVEMENT AND INITIATIVE Responds with constructive actions after manager's feedback. Participates in professional societies. Attempts to keep knowledge of field current. Resourceful in accomplishing tasks. Comments:	Rating: 5 4 3 2 1
8. INNOVATION AND CREATIVITY Generate workable ideas, concepts, and techniques. Willing to attempt new approaches. Simplifies and/or improves procedures, techniques, and processes. Comments:	Rating: 5 4 3 2 1

INTERPERSONAL SKILLS

9. COMMUNICATION Articulates ideas in a clear, concise, and appropriate assertive manner. Produces readable, concise, and accurate written documentation. Provides professional services to both internal and external clients. Comments:	Rating: 5 4 3 2 1
10. SUPERVISION Follows directions and executes plans from program director. Accepts constructive criticism and feedback. Keeps director involved and informed about relevant decisions on a timely basis. Comments:	Rating: 5 4 3 2 1
11. TEAMWORK Assists others when needed. Participates effectively in the work team by offering ideas. Listens to others' suggestions or ideas. Prevents or resolves conflict. Effectively manages team when needed.	Rating: 5 4

| Figure 8.3 | Hospitalist performance evaluation—Format 2 (cont.) |

Comments:	3 2 1
SECTION 5: SUMMARY AND OVERALL EVALUATION	Overall Rating: 5 4 3 2 1
Total Points_____/11 _____Overall Rating	

SECTION 6: FUTURE GOALS AND SUGGESTED IMPROVEMENTS
(Add page if necessary)

SECTION 7: EMPLOYEE COMMENTS
(Add page if necessary)

Approvals

_____   _____   _____   _____
(Name of reviewer/ program director)   Date   *(Name of hospitalist)*   Date

Employee signature acknowledges receipt of review and does not necessarily indicate agreement.

Source: **Brian J. Bossard, MD,** *founder and director, Inpatient Physician Associates, Lincoln, NE.*

Position: Physician Assistant   **Anniversary date:**

Division: Hospitalist Service   **Date of hire:**

5	EXCELLENT	Distinguished performance. Employee consistently and significantly exceeds performance standards.
4	CONSISTENTLY EXCEEDS STANDARDS	Above average performance. Employee consistently achieves and frequently exceeds performance standards.
3	CONSISTENTLY MEETS STANDARDS	Acceptable performance. Employee generally achieves performance standards and maintains a satisfactory performance level in most circumstances.
2	NEEDS IMPROVEMENT	Below average performance. Employee frequently does not achieve a satisfactory performance standard. Improvement is necessary.
1	UNSATISFACTORY	Unacceptable performance. Employee consistently fails to achieve performance standards. Substantial improvement is needed.
NA	NOT APPLICABLE	This rating does not apply to this position.

SECTION I: POSITION-SPECIFIC CRITERIA

Please check the box that most accurately describes employee's performance over the entire period of evaluation.

Criteria:	1	2	3	4	5	N/A
Admits patients referred to *(name of hospitalist service)* under the direction and supervision of attending physician.						
Gathers data (including the history of illness, physical exam, lab tests, and x-rays) for each patient.						
Records patient data in problem-oriented notes using the SOAP format.						
Integrates data into patient database, initiating diagnostic, therapeutic, educational, and dispositional plans under the supervising physician.						
Makes daily rounds on each patient to evaluate needs/progress, adjusting the initial plans, as needed.						
Performs procedures germane to primary patient care.						
Interacts effectively with patients and family.						
	1	2	3	4	5	N/A
Interacts with nursing staff, medical students, and attending physicians around the care of the patient.						
Helps to develop appropriate discharge plans.						

Figure 8.4 — Physician assistant performance evaluation (cont.)

Provides daily voicemail to PCP, when asked.						
Submits patient encounters daily.						
Prepares medical records on a timely basis per hospital requirements.						
Assists in teaching physician assistant or family nurse practitioner students who may rotate through the Inpatient Service.						
Meets all medical staff requirements.						
Attends all required meetings.						
Keeps up with new medical knowledge.						
Maintains patient confidentiality.						
Performs other related duties as assigned by the clinical director or administrative director.						

Comments:

_____

_____

_____

SECTION II: BEHAVIORAL CRITERIA

	1	2	3	4	5
Time management: Employee demonstrates an ability to prioritize work and complete essential tasks in a timely manner. Employee can perform multiple tasks, when necessary, without sacrificing accuracy.					
Judgment: Employee assesses situations from multiple perspectives and appropriately refers concerns to his or her supervisor. Employee uses the appropriate chain of command and makes good decisions under pressure.					
Supports mission: Employee supports the mission of _(name of hospitalist service)_ and acts as a positive role model for fellow employees.					

Figure 8.4

Physician assistant performance evaluation (cont.)

☐ Exceeded expectations for performance

☐ Met expectations; performance is now at an acceptable level

☐ Continues to need improvement

Comments:

_____

_____

_____

SECTION IV: SETTING NEW GOALS

Please identify two or three specific goals for the employee's development during the coming year. Progress toward these goals should be reviewed periodically during the year and at the next annual evaluation meeting. Employees should take an active role in setting goals for their own professional growth and development.

1. _____
   _____
   _____
2. _____
   _____
   _____

Additional comments:

_____

_____

Employee Acknowledgment: My signature verifies that I have seen this evaluation but does not necessarily mean that I agree with my supervisor's assessment of my performance. I understand that I can attach comments to this evaluation if I choose and have those comments become part of my official personnel file in Human Resources.

Employee: _____   **Date:** _____

Supervisor: _____   **Date:** _____

  © 2006 HCPRO, INC. **TOOLS AND STRATEGIES FOR AN EFFECTIVE HOSPITALIST PROGRAM**

Figure 8.4 — Physician assistant performance evaluation (cont.)

	1	2	3	4	5
Adapts to change: Employee adapts to change by willingly learning new policies and procedures. Employee offers constructive suggestions to help improve the program's systems/processes.					
Attitude: Employee displays a positive attitude that reflects belief in teamwork and the importance of supportive working relationships. Treats colleagues, patients, and visitors respectfully.					
Dependability: Employee shows dependability through acceptable attendance and punctuality. Employee shows understanding of the needs of the division when scheduling time off.					
Customer service: Employee practices and promotes high level of service to internal and external customers through timely, accurate and courteous work. Anticipates needs of internal and external customers, where appropriate.					
Accepts constructive criticism: Employee demonstrates willingness to listen to and respond to constructive criticism through positive behavior changes. Does not show defensive behavior during discussion of problem areas.					

Comments:

_____

_____

_____

SECTION III: PROGRESS TOWARD GOALS

In the section below, please describe the progress made toward any goals set at a *previous* introductory or annual evaluation. Briefly describe goals:

Goal: _____

☐ Exceeded expectations for performance

☐ Met expectations; performance is now at an acceptable level

☐ Continues to need improvement

Source: Northeast Inpatient Medical Services, St. Joseph Hospital, Bangor, ME.

Quality improvement and data collection

9

Quality improvement and data collection

Sylvia C. W. McKean, MD, FACP

The role of the hospitalist has evolved beyond demonstrating efficiency of care through length-of-stay reduction to providing enhanced quality of care. Increasingly, competitive markets and pressure from outside agencies—such as the Joint Commission on Accreditation of Healthcare Organizations (JCAHO) and the Agency for Healthcare Research and Quality (AHRQ)—will require hospitals to report performance data.[1,2]

In short order, hospitals in every region of the nation will be compared to one another, and uniform standards will be implemented through public review.[3] To meet emerging standards, hospitals are forming partnerships to pool resources, benchmarking with other institutions, and seeking the expertise of organizations such as the University HealthSystem Consortium (UHC), whose mission is to foster collaboration among academic health centers.[4] In 2006, UHC will begin collecting data to examine how academic health centers employ and financially support hospitalists. In this environment, hospitalists will need to demonstrate improved outcomes relative to their peers. In fact, the performance of hospitalist programs is already being measured, and these programs will be expected to actively set quality parameters, lead teamwork opportunities, and improve performance for individual hospitalists.

Quality measures

The Institute of Medicine (IOM) has categorized quality measures into the following six domains: patient safety, effectiveness, timeliness, patient centeredness, efficiency, and equity.[5] In addition, the National Quality Forum (NQF) has derived the following consensus statements for safety practices that should be universally used in healthcare settings to reduce the risk of harm resulting from processes, systems, or environments[6]:

- **Patient safety measures** include identifying a healthcare proxy, transferring information to all caregivers involved in a patient's care, prominently displaying code status in the patient's chart, assessing risk and prophylaxis for venous thromboembolism, limiting the use of urinary catheters, and avoiding patient falls.

- **Effectiveness of care measures** relate to preoperative cardiac assessment and the use of beta-blockers; prescribing initial antibiotics consistent with current recommendations; assessment and specific medication use for acute coronary syndrome, heart failure, and pneumonia; appropriate vaccinations; and counseling relating to smoking cessation.

- **Timeliness of care measures** include time from hospital admission to arrival on floor, discharge before noon, and time from discharge order to actual discharge.

- **Patient-centeredness measures** are usually based on patient satisfaction surveys.

- **Efficiency of care measures** include length of stay, emergency department visits within 30 days, hospital readmission rate within 30 days, appropriate use of extended-care facilities, use of consultations, and use of tests.

- **Equity of care** requires examination of racial disparities for various quality measures.

All six types of measures are within the purview of hospitalists and are already being measured by many hospitals.

The balanced scorecard

The "balanced scorecard" model is emerging as a strategic framework for action in quality improvement.[4,8,9] By identifying the parameters for measuring quality, any hospitalist service can develop a hospitalist scorecard. The goal is to clarify the vision and strategy of the service by gaining consensus regarding *what* will be measured and *how* the data will be reported.

The Brigham and Women's Hospital (BWH) in Boston has given quality performance measurement a high priority. **Michael Gustafson, MD**, leads the hospital's Center for Clinical Excellence and reports directly to Brigham and Women's chief medical officer.[7] Using data from a balanced scorecard provided by the Center for Clinical Excellence, physicians can track changes—average daily census, discharge volume, etc.—over time (i.e., versus the previous quarter or versus the same quarter in the prior year). The scorecard also enables the Brigham and Women's Faulkner (BWF) Hospitalist Service to analyze quality data (i.e., safety, effectiveness, timeliness, patient-centeredness, efficiency, and equity) from various programs within the service and compare them with data from other practice groups.

Creating a scorecard requires

- setting targets
- aligning strategic initiatives
- allocating resources
- establishing milestones[10]

Once these elements have been established, members of the hospitalist service must be informed and educated about the goals of the initiative, as well as about how rewards will be linked to the performance measures. The balanced scorecard articulates the program's shared vision, supplies strategic feedback "at a glance," and facilitates strategy review and learning.[8,9,10] Ultimately, compensation is linked to strategy as an incentive for corrective action.

The administrative structure of the BWF Hospitalist Service consists of a five-member executive hospitalist strategic council, along with an administrator and a research manager. This body is in charge of strategic planning, development of the balanced scorecard for the BWF Hospitalist Service, and consensus building with the larger group of hospitalists regarding quality improvement and innovation. In collaboration with the Center for Clinical Excellence, **Jeff Schnipper, MD**, director of clinical research for the BWF Hospitalist Service, is responsible for developing the clinical specifications for the hospitalist scorecard with **Amy Bloom, MPH**, the research manager. Given Schnipper's research background and interest in quality improvement, he ensures optimal statistical assessment for accurately profiling the service and the providers. He is also a credible consensus builder for the hospitalist service. The research manager makes sure that the job gets done given competing demands on everyone's time.

The balanced scorecard for the BWF Hospitalist Service is based on the following elements:

1. Recognition of the need to plan for the future

2. Development of a shared vision of what is important for strategic planning

3. Alignment of goals with the goals of BWH and the larger network

4. Empowerment of hospitalists through the executive strategic council leadership

5. Development of "stretch targets" (see the section following this list) through education and open dialogue about the strategy

6. Acceptance of stretch targets by all members of the service

7. Elucidation of strategic initiatives to reach agreed-upon targeted goals

8. Automatic feedback systems using data from the Center for Clinical Excellence and data generated by the research manager

9. Quarterly reassessment and reporting to the department of medicine at BWH

Stretch targets

The establishment and acceptance of stretch targets requires obtaining trustworthy baseline data and developing a consensus of what is attainable if the service is truly committed to improvement. For example, baseline billing data (i.e., the percentage of charges submitted within four days of a patient encounter) are currently being measured for the BWF Hospitalist Service and for individual hospitalists.

After more data become available over a period of time, group and individual targets can be set and incentives can be offered for increasing billing revenue by improving the percentage of charges provided.

Tracking the actual amount of charges per physician is more complex, as billing regulations may change, and linking this data to compensation may provide the wrong incentives (e.g., overcharging for work done, or neglecting nonbillable activities such as providing backup for residents, teaching, and/or performing quality improvements).[11] However, tracking the percentage of charges submitted within a time frame can be easily done through automated billing data already available via Palm Pilot (or other personal digital assistant) billing. Ideally, all members of the service should submit charges 100% of the time for all patient encounters.

Relating compensation to quality of care

The next step is to link compensation (withholds or bonuses, depending on the marketplace) to the established goals. There are pitfalls in relating compensation to quality of care if candidate targets are unattainable or if a performance measure is linked to flawed data. Computer-generated data—while often easier to obtain than data gleaned from chart review—are typically based on data from the discharging physician. Thus, the information may not accurately reflect an individual's performance.

Nevertheless, in keeping with a clearly articulated strategic plan, a hospitalist scorecard facilitates "at a glance" the value of a hospitalist service for hospital administrators and identifies areas that hospitalist leaders might target for improvement. Supplemented with primary care physician (PCP) satisfaction data and chart review of key quality indicators (e.g., transfers to intensive care units and/or readmissions), the hospitalist service can initiate rapid cycle improvements[12] and educational initiatives, the impact of which can be tracked over time.

Generating a hospitalist report card

Using data available from hospital sources is the first step in generating a report card for a hospitalist service. Hospitals have readily accessible financial data, such as average acuity, net operating margin per inpatient discharge, and budget variance and net operating margin per service, as well as efficiency data. In addition, quality measures such as readmission rates, mortality, and intensive care unit transfers are monitored.

Hospitalists may approach the chairman of the department of medicine and hospital administrators for guidance on how to create a report card, the head of health information systems (or head of medical records) for demographic information, and the quality improvement (QI) director for QI data, including JCAHO performance measures.

These leaders should be able to provide specific information about the following:

- Who to approach to find out what data are already being collected
- Who might help examine the data to ensure that they are accurate and allows for meaningful statistical comparison. For example,
  - are physician lists accurate in different comparison groups?
  - what are the response rates relating to patient satisfaction?
  - how many cases/patients are involved in the calculations (mortality and other endpoints)?
  - how is length of stay calculated, how are "outliers" and inter-departmental transfers treated, and how are individual physicians identified?
- Who might advise the service about what data should be measured (i.e., most easily and accurately)?

Even if the data presented are imperfect, it is a critical first step to proactively identify and measure performance quality indicators and set up expectations for improvement.

Once hospitalists determine what parameters are already being measured, the hospitalist service must proactively define quality measures that can be tracked over time and choose the measures that reflect a prioritization of the service's goals. A consensus must be reached on how important each measure is to the specific patient population served by the hospitalist program. A hospitalist service may need to prioritize efficiency, for example, if there are problems relating to average length of stay (ALOS) compared to budgeted ALOS or the ALOS achieved by other physicians on the general medical service.

To supplement quality assessment, hospitalist services may wish to obtain information that is not available through computerized hospital systems. Although it is time consuming, chart review of selected conditions for documentation of patient safety measures (e.g., smoking-cessation counseling, advice for pneumonia patients, evaluation on admission and periodically thereafter for the risk and prevention of pressure ulcers, documentation of information such as left ventricular function in congestive heart failure, and patient/family education) may be already done for the entire department of medicine.

Quality officers should be able to track data according to specific groups for the purposes of comparison. A periodic survey of PCPs for feedback on quality and safety measures may be helpful. Programs can start with a relatively long list of questions and later narrow the list to three to five key questions that the service wishes to track over time and that the busy PCP has time to answer. However, survey response rates from PCPs and/or patients and families will determine the usefulness of the surveys as a quality measurement tools. Ancillary support, such as computer-generated surveys sent to patients after their discharge, or administrative support to mail and collect survey instruments, will be required to generate a meaningful response rate.

Figure 9.1 represents hospitalist operational data and accompanying graphs (average length of stay, diagnosis related group, readmission) from the Hospitalist Program at Ball Memorial Hospital in Muncie, IN. The operation data includes indicators, such as

- discharge time
- readmission percentage
- pre-op totals
- total billed
- admissions
- night float admissions
- total discharges

Figure 9.1   **Hospitalist operational data and graphs**

Total Hospitalist Profile: Acute Inpatient

INDICATOR	Jan-05	Feb-05	Mar-05	Apr-05	May-05	Jun-05	Jul-05	Aug-05	Sep-05	Oct-05	Nov-05	Dec-05	YTD
Volume	356	354	400	391	330	320	340						2491
ALOS A&C	4.7	4.8	4.9	4.9	5.2	5.5	4.7						4.9
ALOS Attending	4.4	4.6	4.7	4.7	5.1	4.9	4.4						4.7
ALOS CM	6.3	5.4	6.6	6.2	7.1	10.1	17.0						6.8
Volume CM	35	138	125	110	93	41	15						542
BMH ALOS	5.7	5.6	5.6	5.8	5.7	5.9	5.7						5.7
Hosp.Deaths													
Hosp. Mortality Rate													
BMH Mortality Rate													
Tot. Overall Mortality Rate- Hospitalists													
Average Age	66	66	68	66	67	69	69						68
BMH Average Age	62	61	61	61	61	61	60						61
BMH Readmission Rate	14.0%	12%	11.5%	10.6%	9%	8%	10%						9.0%
Hosp.Readmission Rate	8.1%	6.2%	8.0%	8.0%	7.0%	7.0%	6.0%						7.2%
ER ONLY/NO ADMIT	6	2	3	1	6	3	2						23
RELEASED FROM CARE EARLY	1	1	2	2	0	0	0						6
Pathway Use	0.0%	2.0%	4.0%	3.6%	3.3%	0.30%	0.30%						2.0%

Individual Physican Profile: Acute Inpatient

INDICATOR	Jan-05	Feb-05	Mar-05	Apr-05	May-05	Jun-05	Jul-05	Aug-05	Sep-05	Oct-05	Nov-05	Dec-05	YTD
Volume	60	57	57	63	59	50	52						398
ALOS	3.7	5.4	4.7	4.7	5.4	4.8	5.1						4.8
Deaths													
Mortality Rate													
Avg Pt Age	68	69	67	65	68	68	69						68
# Readmits	4	3	3	3	4	3	4						24
Readmission Rate	6.7%	5.3%	5.0%	5.0%	7.0%	6%	8%						6.0%
Hosp-Hosp same diagnosis	2	1	0	0	2	1	2						7
Hosp-Hosp different diagnosis	2	2	3	3	2	1	2						14
Pathway Used	0	1	3	1	0	0	0						5
Pathway Use- Alcohol	0	0	0	0	0	0	0						0
Pathway Use- Chest Pain	0	0	0	0	0	0	0						0
Pathway Use- CHF	0	0	0	0	0	0	0						0
Pathway Use- COPD	0	0	0	0	0	0	0						0
Pathway Use- GI	0	1	1	0	0	0	0						2
Pathway Use- Pneumonia	0	0	2	1	0	0	0						3
Pathway Use- Stroke	0	0	0	0	0	0	0						0

Consult/Attending Comparison - QTR. 1,05

INDICATOR	Hospitalist-Attending				Hospitalist-Consulting			
	Jan-05	Feb-05	Mar-05	YTD	Jan-05	Feb-05	Mar-05	YTD
Volume	53	51	49	153	7	6	8	21
ALOS	3.5	5.3	4.5	4.4	5.7	6.3	5.7	5.9
Deaths								
Mortality Rate						-		
Avg Pt Age	68	68	66	67	69	76	79	75

Consult/Attending Comparison - QTR. 2,05

INDICATOR	Hospitalist-Attending				Hospitalist-Consulting			
	Apr-05	May-05	Jun-05	YTD	Apr-05	May-05	Jun-05	YTD
Volume	57	49	40	299	6	10	10	47
ALOS	4.7	5.3	4.8	4.7	5	5.8	5	5.5
Deaths								
Mortality Rate								
Avg Pt Age	65	67	66	66	71	74	77	74

Consult/Attending Comparison - QTR. 3,05

INDICATOR	Hospitalist-Attending				Hospitalist-Consulting			
	Jul-05	Aug-05	Sep-05	YTD	Jul-05	Aug-05	Sep-05	YTD
Volume	46			345	6			53
ALOS	4.3			4.6	11.2			6.1
Deaths								
Mortality Rate								
Avg Pt Age	69			67	69			74

Consult/Attending Comparison - QTR. 4,05

INDICATOR	Hospitalist-Attending				Hospitalist-Consulting			
	Oct-05	Nov-05	Dec-05	YTD	Oct-05	Nov-05	Dec-05	YTD
Volume								
ALOS								
Deaths								
Mortality Rate								
Avg Pt Age								

Source: Jeffery R. Dichter, MD; Partner, Medical Consultants PC, Muncie, IN; Founder of the Hospital Medicine Program at Ball Memorial Hospital, Muncie, IN.

Figure 9.1 — Hospitalist operational data and graphs (cont.)

Hospitalist Rehab Profile

INDICATOR	Jan-05	Feb-05	Mar-05	Apr-05	May-05	Jun-05	Jul-05	Aug-05	Sep-05	Oct-05	Nov-05	Dec-05	YTD
Volume-Total	13	14	11	8	7	14	11						78
Volume- MD 1	2	1	1	0	0	2	0						6
Vol-MD2	0	2	2	0	0	0	0						4
Vol-MD3	0	2	2	3	0	4	3						14
Vol-MD4	2	2	0	1	1	4	2						12
Vol-MD5	4	3	1	0	1	1	1						11
Vol-MD6	1	1	2	2	2	0	1						9
Vol-MD7	1	3	2	1	3	2	1						13
Vol- MD8	3	0	1	1	0	1	0						6
ALOS-Total	8.7	7.1	10.0	7.9	10.1	8.3	8.4						8.5
ALOS- MD1	7.5	11.0	7.0	0.0	0.0	10.5	0.0						9.0
ALOS-MD2	0	6	11	0	0	0	4						6.4
ALOS-MD3	0	8	15	6	0	7	17						10.0
ALOS-MD4	6.5	5	0	9	13	7.2	6						7.2
ALOS-MD5	10	8.7	21	0	9	6	8						10
ALOS-MD6	7.0	5.0	5.0	9.0	7.5	0.0	3.0						6.4
ALOS-MD7	14	6.7	6	3	11.3	7	7						8
ALOS- MD8	6	0	10	16	0	19	0						10.5
Deaths	0	0	0	0	0	0	0						0
Mortality Rate	0.0%	0.0%	0.0%	0.0%	0.0%	0.0%	0.0%						0.0%
Average Age	75	75	71	66	65	73	79						73
Av.Age-MD1	67	70	61	0	0	65	0						66
Av.Age-MD2	0	65	59	0	0	0	89						74
Av.Age-MD3	0	76	75	72	0	80	68						74
Av.Age-MD4	84	76	0	79	79	74	87						79
Av.Age-MD5	71	78	78	0	60	86	77						74
Av.Age-MD6	83	79	77	66	65	0	70						72
Av. Age-MD7	79	0	77	48	0	78	0						73
Av.Age-MD8	70	77	73	51	62	71	79						70

Hospitalist TCU Profile

INDICATOR	Jan-05	Feb-05	Mar-05	Apr-05	May-05	Jun-05	Jul-05	Aug-05	Sep-05	Oct-05	Nov-05	Dec-05	YTD
Volume-Total	27	35	51	40	29	19	24						225
Vol-MD1	0	0	1	1	0	0	0						2
Vol-MD2	0	2	7	6	4	1	4						24
Vol-MD3	2	11	8	6	1	1	5						34
Vol-MD4	2	3	6	4	8	9	5						37
Vol-MD5	11	7	17	0	3	0	3						38
Vol-MD6	3	5	9	10	1	4	3						35
Vol-MD7	4	7	1	3	10	2	4						31
Vol- MD8	5	0	5	10	2	2	0						24
ALOS-Total	12.0	9.0	9.3	10.4	9.0	9.2	0.0						9.8
ALOS-MD1	0.0	0.0	2.0	15.0	0.0	0.0	0.0						8.5
ALOS-MD2	0.0	13.0	9.6	13.0	7.7	7.0	10.7						10.5
ALOS-MD3	9.5	9.1	11.4	10.1	12.0	10.0	11.2						10.2
ALOS-MD4	17.0	13.0	10.8	11.2	10.6	10.6	16.0						12.0
ALOS-MD5	9.5	17.6	10.6	0.0	15.7	0.0	8.0						11.8
ALOS-MD6	26.0	5.0	6.6	10.0	43.0	10.5	11.3						10.9
ALOS-MD7	13.5	13.3	17.0	11.6	12.5	17.5	13.5						13.3
ALOS- MD8	19.2	0.0	8.2	11.8	21.0	10.0	0.0						13.2

Source: Jeffery R. Dichter, MD; Partner, Medical Consultants PC, Muncie, IN; Founder of the Hospital Medicine Program at Ball Memorial Hospital, Muncie, IN.

Figure 9.1 — Hospitalist operational data and graphs (cont.)

	Jan-05	Feb-05	Mar-05	Apr-05	May-05	Jun-05	Jul-05	Aug-05	Sep-05	Oct-05	Nov-05	Dec-05	YTD
Deaths													
Mortality Rate													
Mortality Rate-MD1													
Mortality Rate-MD2													
Mortality Rate-MD3													
Mortality Rate-MD4													
Mortality Rate-MD5													
Mortality Rate-MD6													
Mortality Rate-MD7													
Mortality Rate- MD8													
Av.Age-MD1	0	0	89	86	0	0	0.0%						87
Av.Age-MD2	0	78	75	74	76	87	74						75
Av. Age MD3	80	81	79	73	76	84	84						79
Av.Age-MD4	81	80	80	71	73	78	78						77
Av.Age-MD5	76	81	81	0	68	0	81						78
Av.Age-MD6	87	75	79	77	75	66	76						77
Av. Age- MD7	76	0	82	71	73	84	76						75
Av.Age-MD8	79	73	82	78	75	79	0						75

Hospitalist Discharge Disposition Rate w/ Comparison Profile- Indicator Change

INDICATOR	Jan-05	Feb-05	Mar-05	Apr-05	May-05	Jun-05	Jul-05	Aug-05	Sep-05	Oct-05	Nov-05	Dec-05	YTD
Hosp.AMA	1.5%	0.5%	0.4%	0.4%	0.5%	0.0%	0.5%						0.6%
Hosp.Home/HHC	7.9%	8.2%	10.8%	10.9%	16.5%	9.7%	11.6%						11.3%
Hosp.Home	61.0%	67.3%	60.4%	66.8%	59.0%	68.0%	65.6%						63.4%
Hosp.ICF	0.5%	0.0%	0.0%	0.4%	0.0%	0.0%	0.5%						0.3%
Hosp. SNF	29.0%	24.0%	28.3%	21.4%	24.0%	22.3%	21.7%						24.5%
BMH AMA	0.6%	1.3%	1.0%	0.3%	1.0%	0.5%	1.4%						0.6%
BMH Home/HHC	3.7%	2.8%	3.0%	1.4%	1.7%	2.2%	2.8%						2.1%
BMH Home	55.0%	58.0%	59.0%	60.0%	64.0%	59.0%	57.0%						55.0%
BMH ICF	0.2%	0.2%	0.7%	0.3%	0.3%	0.3%	0.1%						0.2%
BMH SNF	16.0%	12.9%	12.7%	11.6%	10.1%	10.1%	10.2%						11.8%

Source: Jeffery R. Dichter, MD; Partner, Medical Consultants PC, Muncie, IN; Founder of the Hospital Medicine Program at Ball Memorial Hospital, Muncie, IN.

Figure 9.1 **Hospitalist operational data and graphs (cont.)**

Hospitalist - Comp/ALOS by Payor 2005

INDICATOR	Jan-05	Feb-05	Mar-05	Apr-05	May-05	Jun-05	Jul-05	Aug-05	Sep-05	Oct-05	Nov-05	Dec-05	YTD
Hosp. BC	4	5	5	4.8	5.6	5.4	3.7						4.8
Hosp.Commercial	3.8	4.6	3.5	4.3	3.2	7.3	4.3						4.3
Hosp.MCCD	5.1	7.1	5.2	6.7	4.4	9.1	5.7						6
Hosp. Medicare	5.8	5.3	6.2	6	6.4	5.9	6						5.9
Hosp.Self Pay	6	0	0	0	0	0	4						5.9
Hosp. WC	0	3	0	0	0	1	1						2.7
BMH BC	4.9	4	5	5.5	4.9	5.9	5						5
BMH Commercial	4.9	4.7	4.8	4.3	4.8	4.6	4.6						4.6
BMH MCCD	6.7	5.8	6	5.7	6.4	6.4	5.5						6
BMH Medicare	6.2	6.4	6.2	6.7	6	6.7	6.3						6.4
BMH Self Pay	3.3	0	3.4	3.7	3.7	3	4.9						3.8
BMH WC	1	6	3	3.3	1	2.7	3.3						3.4

Hospitalist SI/IS Profile

INDICATOR	Jan-05	Feb-05	Mar-05	Apr-05	May-05	Jun-05	Jul-05	Aug-05	Sep-05	Oct-05	Nov-05	Dec-05	YTD
Avoidable Days- MD1	0	0	0	0	0	0	0						0
Avoidable Days- MD2	0	1	0	1	1	0	2						5
Avoidable Days Rate-MD2	0.0%	1.3%	0%	1.1%	0.4%	0.0%	1.6%						0.7%
Inappropriate Admit-MD2	0	0	0	0	0	0	0						0
Inappropriate TOB Admit-MD2	0	0	0	1	0	0	0						1
Avoidable Days-MD3	0	1	0	0	2	2	0						5
Avoidable Days Rate-MD3	0.0%	0.0%	0.0%	0.0%	0.3%	0.8%	0.0%						0.2%
Inappropriate Admit-MD3	0	0	0	1	0	0	0						1
Inappropriate TOB Admit-MD3	0	0	0	0	0	0	0						0
Avoidable Days- MD4	0	0	0	0	0	1	0						1
Avoidable Days Rate-MD4	0.0%	0.0%	0.0%	0.0%	0.0%	1.1%	0.0%						0.2%
Inappropriate Admit-MD4	0	0	0	0	0	0	0						0
Inappropriate TOB Admit-MD4	0	0	0	0	0	0	0						0
Avoidable Days-MD5	0	1	0	0	0	1	1						3
Avoidable Days Rate-MD5	0.0%	0.4%	0.0%	0.0%	0.0%	1.2%	2.1%						0.5%
Inappropriate Admit-MD5	0	1	0	0	0	0	0						1
Inappropriate TOB Admit-MD5	0	0	0	0	0	0	0						0
Avoidable Days-MD6	0	0	0	0	0	2	0						2
Avoidable Days Rate-MD6	0.0%	0.0%	0.0%	0.0%	0.0%	0.9%	0.0%						0.2%
Inappropriate Admit-MD6	0	0	0	0	0	0	0						0
Inappropriate TOB Admit-MD6	0	0	0	0	0	0	0						0
Avoidable Days-MD7	0	1	2	4	1	1	0						9
Avoidable Days Rate-MD7	0	0.8%	1.4%	1.4%	0.0%	0.4%	0.0%						1.0%
Inappropriate Admit-MD7	0	0	0	1	0	0	0						1
Inappropriate TOB Admit-MD7	0	0	0	0	0	0	0						0
Avoidable Days-MD8	2	2	0	2	1	1	0						8
Avoidable Days Rate-MD8	1.5%	1.7%	0.0%	2.1%	0.8%	0.3%	0.0%						1.0%
Inappropriate Admit-MD8	2	1	0	0	0	0	0						3
Inappropriate TOB Admit-MD8	0	0	0	0	0	0	0						0

Source: Jeffery R. Dichter, MD; Partner, Medical Consultants PC, Muncie, IN; Founder of the Hospital Medicine Program at Ball Memorial Hospital, Muncie, IN.

Figure 9.1   Hospitalist operational data and graphs (cont.)

Operational Data

Indicator	Jan-05	Feb-05	Mar-05	Apr-05	May-05	Jun-05	Jul-05	Aug-05	Sep-05	Oct-05	Nov-05	Dec-05
Discharge time	11:09	11:58	12:20	11:04	11:26	12:22	11:28					
Group Volume	275	287	356	276	227	220	292					
Group Re-Admit Percentage	8%	6%	8%	8%	7%	8%	6%					
Pre-Op Totals	12	22	24	22	22	13	14					
Total Billed	1985	1888	2184	2156	2122	1738	1968					
Average Daily	18	15	18	19	16.6	17	16					
Group admissions	356	354	399	389	330	186	205					
Group night census	162	160	174	165	167	156	146					
Group Discharges	274	287	356	275	189	198	296					

Operational Data- Hospitalist 1

Indicator	Jan-05	Feb-05	Mar-05	Apr-05	May-05	Jun-05	Jul-05	Aug-05	Sep-05	Oct-05	Nov-05	Dec-05
Discharge time	10:48	10:15	10:09	10:00	10:34	10:06	10:11					
Volume for D/C	43	48	47	67	28	54	40					
Re-Admit %	7%	6%	6%	5%	7%	6%	8%					
Pre-Op Totals	2	3	4	4	2	2	1					
Total Billed	313	301	267	433	282	370	253					
Average Daily	20	17	18	19	17	19	17					
Admissions	41	32	27	35	44	35	27					
Night Float Admissions	14	16	36	0	41	25	29					
Total Discharges	43	47	47	67	28	54	40					

Operational Data- Hospitalist 2

Indicator	Jan-05	Feb-05	Mar-05	Apr-05	May-05	Jun-05	Jul-05	Aug-05	Sep-05	Oct-05	Nov-05	Dec-05
Discharge time	10:28	11:40	11:14	10:03	10:15	10:37	10:53					
Volume for D/C	61	55	59	38	38	51	57					
Re-Admit %	8%	6%	4%	4%	9%	7%	4%					
Pre-Op Totals	4	2	5	3	3	3	2					
Total Billed	329	272	301	272	308	420	414					
Average Daily	14	13	19	18	14	17	17					
Admissions	33	28	34	41	35	46	44					
Night Float Admissions	0	19	13	41	0	0	0					
Total Discharges	58	53	59	38	34	51	56					

Source: Jeffery R. Dichter, MD; Partner, Medical Consultants PC, Muncie, IN; Founder of the Hospital Medicine Program at Ball Memorial Hospital, Muncie, IN.

Figure 9.1 | Hospitalist operational data and graphs (cont.)

Operational Data- Hospitalist 3

Indicator	Jan-05	Feb-05	Mar-05	Apr-05	May-05	Jun-05	Jul-05	Aug-05	Sep-05	Oct-05	Nov-05	Dec-05
Discharge time	10:57	12:10	12:25	11:56	11:36	11:49	12:12					
Volume for D/C	20	43	50	56	18	11	47					
Re-Admit %	9%	9%	12%	14%	9%	7%	3%					
Pre-Op Totals	0	5	6	7	0	0	3					
Total Billed	172	320	376	434	215	181	352					
Average Daily	17	13	17	18	17	16	16					
Admissions	23	16	25	33	16	21	39					
Night Float Admissions	52	0	0	0	33	0	41					
Total Discharges	25	43	50	56	11	2	47					

Operational Data- Hospitalist 4

Indicator	Jan-05	Feb-05	Mar-05	Apr-05	May-05	Jun-05	Jul-05	Aug-05	Sep-05	Oct-05	Nov-05	Dec-05
Discharge time	12:12	12:15	11:40	11:09	11:32	12:30	12:35					
Volume for D/C	16	37	47	28	36	41	35					
Re-Admit %	8%	6%	7%	8%	4%	2%	8%					
Pre-Op Totals	1	6	4	1	6	4	0					
Total Billed	160	297	279	245	290	320	234					
Average Daily	16	14	15	22	17	17	14					
Admissions	17	35	45	20	36	35	38					
Night Float Admissions	96	0	42	3	36	28	44					
Total Discharges	15	34	43	27	25	40	40					

Operational Data- Hospitalist 5

Indicator	Jan-05	Feb-05	Mar-05	Apr-05	May-05	Jun-05	Jul-05	Aug-05	Sep-05	Oct-05	Nov-05	Dec-05
Discharge time	11:12	11:10	11:39	11:22	11:31	12:38	11:28					
Volume for D/C	80	38	54	30	16	11	67					
Re-Admit %	4%	5%	4%	9%	13%	0%	3%					
Pre-Op Totals	4	2	4	5	1	0	5					
Total Billed	512	236	359	313	152	144	432					
Average Daily	20	17	21	18	12	12	17					
Admissions	48	31	21	38	7	18	26					
Night Float Admissions	0	42	30	0	57	21	5					
Total Discharges	81	38	54	30	15	9	64					

Source: Jeffery R. Dichter, MD; Partner, Medical Consultants PC, Muncie, IN; Founder of the Hospital Medicine Program at Ball Memorial Hospital, Muncie, IN.

Figure 9.1 — Hospitalist operational data and graphs (cont.)

Operational Data- Hospitalist 6

Indicator	Jan-05	Feb-05	Mar-05	Apr-05	May-05	Jun-05	Jul-05	Aug-05	Sep-05	Oct-05	Nov-05	Dec-05
Discharge time	10:54	11:58	11:01	10:28	11:17	10:40	11:26					
Volume for D/C	38	40	44	18	57	21	46					
Re-Admit %	9%	7%	17%	5%	3%	13%	8%					
Pre-Op Totals	1	4	1	2	7	2	3					
Total Billed	359	239	301	157	527	235	283					
Average Daily	19	18	20	16	22	17	16					
Admissions	36	32	30	20	30	17	31					
Night Float Admissions	0	51	0	103	0	21	30					
Total Discharges	28	40	48	8	50	17	46					

Operational Data- Hospitalist 7

Indicator	Jan-05	Feb-05	Mar-05	Apr-05	May-05	Jun-05	Jul-05	Aug-05	Sep-05	Oct-05	Nov-05	Dec-05
Discharge time	12:52	12:58	3:30	1:12	1:15	1:38						
Volume for D/C	17	26	55	39	34	16						
Re-Admit %	7%	6%	9%	5%	4%	14%						
Pre-Op Totals	0	0	0	0	0	0						
Total Billed	140	223	301	302	348	68						
Average Daily	17	15	18	19	17	23						
Admissions	12	25	26	21	28	25						
Night Float Admissions	0	32	53	34	0	61						
Total Discharges	17	25	55	39	26	25						

Source: Jeffery R. Dichter, MD; Partner, Medical Consultants PC, Muncie, IN; Founder of the Hospital Medicine Program at Ball Memorial Hospital, Muncie, IN.

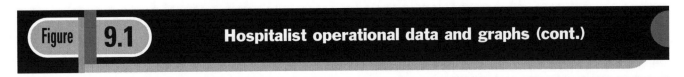

Figure 9.1 Hospitalist operational data and graphs (cont.)

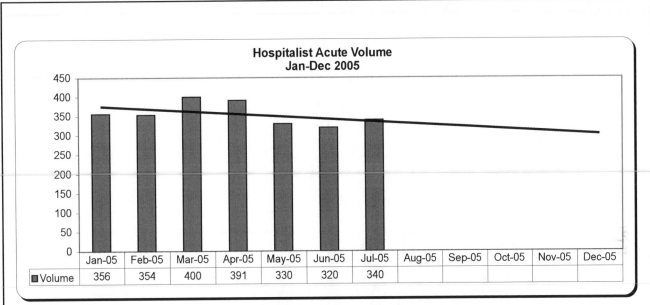

Hospitalist Acute Volume
Jan-Dec 2005

	Jan-05	Feb-05	Mar-05	Apr-05	May-05	Jun-05	Jul-05	Aug-05	Sep-05	Oct-05	Nov-05	Dec-05
■Volume	356	354	400	391	330	320	340					

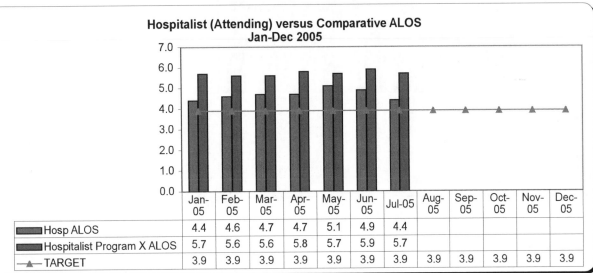

Hospitalist (Attending) versus Comparative ALOS
Jan-Dec 2005

	Jan-05	Feb-05	Mar-05	Apr-05	May-05	Jun-05	Jul-05	Aug-05	Sep-05	Oct-05	Nov-05	Dec-05
Hosp ALOS	4.4	4.6	4.7	4.7	5.1	4.9	4.4					
Hospitalist Program X ALOS	5.7	5.6	5.6	5.8	5.7	5.9	5.7					
TARGET	3.9	3.9	3.9	3.9	3.9	3.9	3.9	3.9	3.9	3.9	3.9	3.9

Source: Jeffery R. Dichter, MD; Partner, Medical Consultants PC, Muncie, IN; Founder of the Hospital Medicine Program at Ball Memorial Hospital, Muncie, IN.

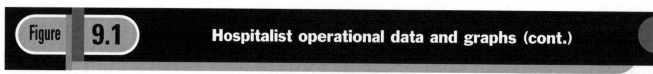

Figure 9.1   Hospitalist operational data and graphs (cont.)

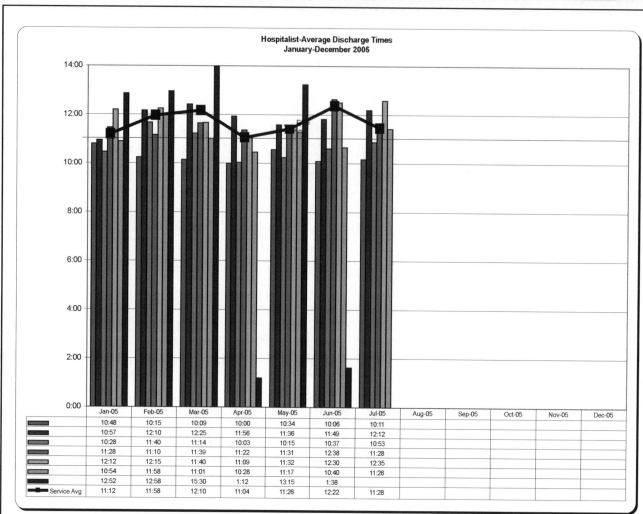

	Jan-05	Feb-05	Mar-05	Apr-05	May-05	Jun-05	Jul-05	Aug-05	Sep-05	Oct-05	Nov-05	Dec-05
	10:48	10:15	10:09	10:00	10:34	10:06	10:11					
	10:57	12:10	12:25	11:56	11:36	11:49	12:12					
	10:28	11:40	11:14	10:03	10:15	10:37	10:53					
	11:28	11:10	11:39	11:22	11:31	12:38	11:28					
	12:12	12:15	11:40	11:09	11:32	12:30	12:35					
	10:54	11:58	11:01	10:28	11:17	10:40	11:26					
	12:52	12:58	15:30	1:12	13:15	1:38						
Service Avg	11:12	11:58	12:10	11:04	11:26	12:22	11:28					

Source: Jeffery R. Dichter, MD; Partner, Medical Consultants PC, Muncie, IN; Founder of the Hospital Medicine Program at Ball Memorial Hospital, Muncie, IN.

Figure 9.1 Hospitalist operational data and graphs (cont.)

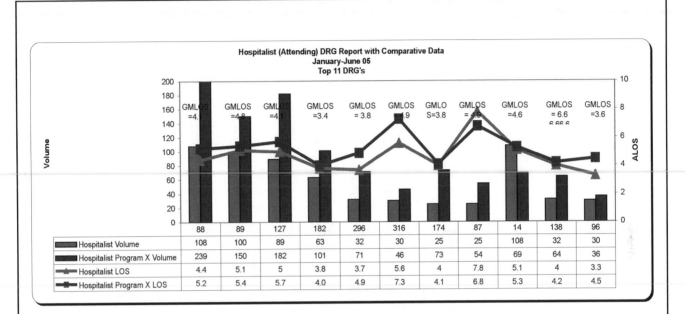

Source: Jeffery R. Dichter, MD; Partner, Medical Consultants PC, Muncie, IN; Founder of the Hospital Medicine Program at Ball Memorial Hospital, Muncie, IN.

Figure **9.1** Hospitalist operational data and graphs (cont.)

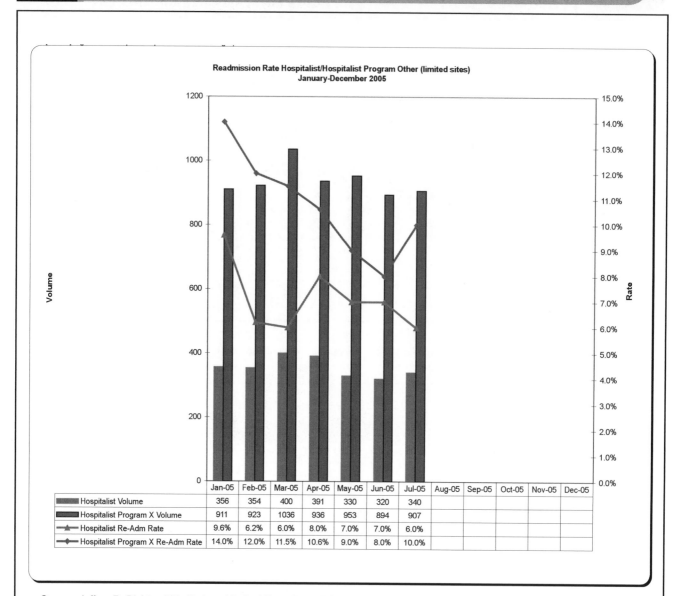

Source: Jeffery R. Dichter, MD; Partner, Medical Consultants PC, Muncie, IN; Founder of the Hospital Medicine Program at Ball Memorial Hospital, Muncie, IN.

Figure 9.2 represents a snapshot of an operation data scorecard for from the hospitalist program at Ball Memorial Hospital in Muncie, IN. It measures the following factors for both the group and individual hospitalists:

- Discharge time
- Readmission percentage
- Pre-op totals
- Total billed encounters
- Average daily census
- Total admissions
- Night float admissions
- Total discharges

Figure 9.3 demonstrates an example of a hospitalist report card and accompanying data derived using Centers for Medicare & Medicaid Services/National Quality Improvement/the JCAHO ORYX measures. The data come from Inpatient Physician Associates, which serves BryanLGH Medical Center in Lincoln, NE.

Frequency of reports

A hospitalist service might incorporate the report card into quarterly reports generated for senior physician leadership and therefore might want to prioritize performance measures based on the overall strategic goals of the larger organization. For example, if the hospital has a very high census, earlier discharge times and decreased ALOS are critical to the efficiency and bottom line of the hospital and to avoiding emergency room diversion.

If third-party payers have negotiated specific quality measures (e.g., diabetes control), the hospitalist service might select a performance measure that tracks the management of diabetes in the hospital—such as the percentage of glucose test values smaller than a defined value or the percentage of patients who had a laboratory test of diabetic control, the HgAIC, measured within the past three months. Quarterly reports also should document innovative new programs or pilots initiated by the hospitalist service. Dedicated administrative support is needed to generate timely, actionable quarterly reports.

Figure 9.4 is a template of a quarterly report submitted to the hospital administration at Brigham and Women's Hospital made possible by the assistance of Lance Rachelefsky, hospital administrator for the BWF Hospitalist Service.

Figure 9.2   **Operational data snapshot**

Operational data 2005:
Group profile

Key:
D/C = Discharge

Month	January	February	March	April	May	June	July	August
D/C time	11:09am	11:58am	12:20pm	11:04am	11:26am	12:22pm	11:28am	**11:28am**
Group volume for D/C	275	287	356	276	227	220	292	**302**
Group readmit %	8%	6%	8%	8%	7%	6%	6%	**6%**
Pre-op totals	12	22	24	22	22	13	14	**15**
Total billed encounters	1985	1888	2184	2156	2122	1738	1968	**1902**
Average daily census	18	15	18	19	16.6	17	16	**13**
Group admissions	356	354	399	389	330	186	205	**242**
Group night census	162	160	174	165	167	156	146	**125**
Group discharges	274	287	356	275	189	198	296	**302**

Notes:
D/C time is derived from the group volume
Total number of pre-ops is for the entire group
Billed encounters are those submitted to the billing department
Group night census is for the entire month

Operational data 2005:
Individual hospitalists

Hospitalist 1

Month	January	February	March	April	May	June	July	August	
D/C time	10:48am	10:15am	10:09am	10:00am	10:34am	10:06am	10:11am	**9:45am**	
Volume for D/C		43	48	47	67	28	54	40	53
Readmit %	4/60 = 7%	3/57 = 6%	3/57 = 6%	3/62 = 5%	4/59 = 7%	3/50 = 6%	4/52 = 8%	**6/53 =11%**	
Total pre-ops		2	3	4	4	2	2	1	3
Total billed encounters		313	301	267	433	282	370	253	280
Average daily census		20	17	18	19	17	19	17	11
Admissions		41	32	27	35	44	35	27	38
Night float admits		14	16	36	0	41	25	29	0
Total discharges		43	47	47	67	28	54	40	53

Hospitalist 2

Month	January	February	March	April	May	June	July	August	
D/C time	10:28am	11:40am	11:14am	10:03am	10:15am	10:37am	10:53am	**9:53am**	
Volume for D/C		61	55	59	38	38	51	57	44
Readmit %	5/59 =8%	3/48 = 6%	2/53 =4%	3/68 = 4%	4/45 = 9%	4/60 = 7%	3/71 = 4%	**1/51 = 2%**	
Total pre-ops		4	2	5	3	3	3	2	4
Total billed encounters		329	272	301	272	308	420	414	281
Average daily census		14	13	19	18	14	17	17	13
Admissions		33	28	34	41	35	46	44	35
Night float admits		0	19	13	41	0	0	0	25
Total discharges		58	53	59	38	34	51	56	44

Figure 9.2 Operational data snapshot (cont.)

Hospitalist 3

Month	January	February	March	April	May	June	July	August
D/C time	10:57am	12:10pm	12:25pm	11:56am	11:36am	11:49am	12:12	**11:42am**
Volume for D/C	20	43	50	56	18	11	47	**52**
Readmit %	4/42 = 9%	4/44 = 9%	5/41=12%	5/37=14%	4/44 = 9%	1/15 = 7%	2/59 = 3%	**2/51 = 4%**
Total pre-ops	0	5	6	7	0	0	3	**0**
Total billed encounters	172	320	376	434	215	181	352	**324**
Average daily census	17	13	17	18	17	16	16	**15**
Admissions	23	16	25	33	16	21	39	**40**
Night float admits	52	0	0	0	33	0	41	**25**
Total discharges	25	43	50	56	11	2	47	**41**

Hospitalist 4

Month	January	February	March	April	May	June	July	August
D/C time	12:12pm	12:15pm	11:40am	11:09am	11:32am	12:30pm	12:35	**11:59am**
Volume for D/C	16	37	47	28	36	41	35	**39**
Readmit %	4/48 =8%	3/48 = 6%	4/54 = 7%	5/38 =13%	2/48 = 4%	1/45 = 2%	4/48 = 8%	**2/49 = 4%**
Total pre-ops	1	6	4	1	6	4	0	**4**
Total billed encounters	160	297	279	245	290	320	234	**265**
Average daily census	16	14	15	22	17	17	14	**13**
Admissions	17	35	45	20	36	35	38	**30**
Night float admits	96	0	42	3	36	28	44	**17**
Total discharges	15	34	43	27	25	40	40	**39**

Hospitalist 5

Month	January	February	March	April	May	June	July	August
D/C time	11:12am	11:10am	11:39am	11:22am	11:31am	12:38am	11:28am	**11:17am**
Volume for D/C	80	38	54	30	16	11	67	**43**
Readmit %	3/70 = 4%	3/55 = 5%	3/71 = 4%	4/47= 9%	4/30 = 13%	0/0	2/59 = 3%	**2/46 = 4%**
Total pre-ops	4	2	4	5	1	0	5	**0**
Total billed encounters	512	236	359	313	152	144	432	**289**
Average daily census	20	17	21	18	12	12	17	**14**
Admissions	48	31	21	38	7	18	26	**30**
Night float admits	0	42	30	0	57	21	5	**30**
Total discharges	81	38	54	30	15	9	64	**30**

 © 2006 HCPRO, INC.

Figure 9.2 — **Operational data snapshot (cont.)**

Hospitalist 6

Month	January	February	March	April	May	June	July	August
D/C time	10:54am	11:58am	11:01am	10:28am	11:17am	10:40am	11:26am	**10:49**
Volume for D/C	38	40	44	18	57	21	46	**44**
Readmit %	5/46 =11%	4/58 = 7%	8/48=17%	3/58=5%	3/57 = 3%	4/32 = 13	4/49 = 8%	**7/47 = 15%**
Total pre-ops	1	4	1	2	7	2	3	**1**
Total billed encounters	359	239	301	157	527	235	283	**273**
Average daily census	19	18	20	16	22	17	16	**15**
Admissions	36	32	30	20	30	17	31	**39**
Night float admits	0	51	0	102	0	21	30	**28**
Total discharges	28	40	48	8	50	17	46	**43**

Hospitalist 7

Month	January	February	March	April	May	June	July	August
D/C time	12:52pm	12:58pm	3:30pm	1:12pm	1:15pm	1:38pm	X	
Volume for D/C	17	26	55	39	34	16	X	
Readmit %	4/28 =14%	2/36 = 6%	6/66 =9%	3/58 = 5%	2/45 = 4%	5/36 = 14	X	
Total pre-ops	0	0	0	0	0	0	X	
Total billed encounters	140	223	301	302	348	68	X	
Average daily census	17	15	18	19	17	23	X	
Admissions	12	25	26	21	28	25	X	
Night float admits	0	32	53	34	0	61	X	
Total discharges	17	25	55	39	26	25	X	

Source: **Jeffery R. Dichter, MD;** Partner, Medical Consultants PC, Muncie, IN; Founder of the Hospital Medicine Program at Ball Memorial Hospital, Muncie, IN.

© 2006 HCPro, Inc. TOOLS AND STRATEGIES FOR AN EFFECTIVE HOSPITALIST PROGRAM

Figure 9.3 — Hospitalist report—Pneumonia core measures initiative

PNEUMONIA

CMS Inpatient National Quality Improvement Project—Selected ORYX Report Definitions

PN-1 Oxygenation assessment: Documentation that pneumonia patients had an assessment an assessment of arterial oxygenation by arterial blood gas measurement or pulse oximetry within 24 hours prior to or after arrival at the hospital

Included Populations:

- All PN patients with physician documentation of the diagnosis of pneumonia written before or at the time of admission including patients transferred from long-term care facilities

Excluded Populations:

- Patients received in transfer from another acute care or critical access hospital, including another facility's emergency department
- Patients who have no working diagnosis of pneumonia at the time of admission
- Patients receiving Comfort Measures Only
- Patients less than 18 years of age

PN-2 Pneumococcal vaccination: Documentation that patients age 65 years of age or older were screened for pneumococcal vaccine status [and the vaccination?] was administered to inpatients during this admission, unless given prior to admission, patient refused, or allergy or sensitivity is documented

Included Populations:

- All PN patients with physician documentation of the diagnosis of pneumonia written before or at the time of admission including patients transferred from long-term care facilities

Excluded Populations:

- Patients received in transfer from another acute care or critical access hospital, including another emergency department
- Patients who left against medical advice
- Patients who have no working diagnosis of pneumonia at the time of admission
- Patients receiving Comfort Measures Only
- Patients less than 65 years of age
- Expired patients
- Patients who were discharged to hospice care
- Patients who were transferred to another short-term general hospital for inpatient care
- Patients who were discharged to a federal hospital

PN-3 Blood cultures: Documentation that a blood culture was collected before the first dose of antibiotic was administered in the hospital, 3a captures cultures that were done prior to admission as well as after, 3b is only in-hospital

Included Populations:

- All PN patients with physician documentation of the diagnosis of pneumonia written before or at the time of admission including patients transferred from long-term care facilities

Excluded Populations:

- Patients received in transfer from another acute care or critical access hospital
- Patients who have no working diagnosis of pneumonia at the time of admission
- Patients receiving Comfort Measures only
- Patients less than 18 years of age
- Patients for whom a blood culture was not obtained

PN-4 Adult smoking cessation advice/counseling: Documentation that the adult patient 18 years of age and older has smoked cigarettes anytime during the year prior to hospital arrival and received cessation advice/counseling during the hospital stay

Included Populations:

- All PN patients with physician documentation of the diagnosis of pneumonia written before or at the time of admission including patients transferred from long-term care facilities

Excluded Populations:

- Patients transferred to another acute care hospital
- Patients who left against medical advice
- Patients discharged to hospice
- Expired patients
- Patients who have no working diagnosis of pneumonia at the time of admission
- Patients receiving Comfort Measures only
- Patients less than 18 years of age
- Patients transferred to a federal hospital
- Patients received in transfers from another hospital's emergency department

PN-5 Antibiotic timing: Timeliness of antibiotic administration for pneumonia inpatients: PN5 refers to mean/average time of cases, PN5b refers to percent of cases meeting the K51 4-hour goal

Included Populations:

- All PN patients with physician documentation of the diagnosis of pneumonia written before or at the time of admission including patients transferred from long-term care facilities

Excluded Populations:

- Patients received in transfer from another acute care hospital, including another emergency department
- Patients who have no working diagnosis of pneumonia at the time of admission
- Patients receiving Comfort Measures Only
- Patients less than 18 years of age
- Patients whose initial antibiotic was administered more than 36 hours from the time of arrival
- Patients who did not receive antibiotics during hospitalization
- Patients who have received antibiotics within 24 hours prior to hospital arrival

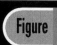

Figure 9.3 — Hospitalist report—Pneumonia core measures initiative (cont.)

PN-6 Initial antibiotic selection for immunocompetent patients:
Immunocompetent patients with pneumonia who receive an initial antibiotic regimen during the first 24 hours consistent with current guidelines (6a & 6b combined)

PN-6a Initial antibiotic selection for immunocompetent patients ICU:
ICU pneumonia patients who received an initial antibiotic regimen consistent with current guidelines during the first 24 hours of their hospitalization

Included Populations:

- All ICU patients including patients transferred from long-term care facilities on the following antibiotics:
    - IV -lactam (ceftriaxone, cefotaxime, ampicillin-sulbactam) plus IV macrolide (erythromycin, azithromycin) or IV -lactam plus IV quinolone
    - If documented -lactam allergy: IV quinolone plus IV clindamycin or IV quinolone plus IV vancomycin
- For patients with pseudomonal risk (bronchiectasis or malnutrition documented at time of admission or serum albumin less than 3.0 within the first 24 hours after hospital arrival) the following antibiotics should be used:
    - IV antipseudomonal -lactam (cefepime, imipenem, meropenem, piperacillin-tozobactam) plus IV antipseudomonal quinolone (ciprofloxacin, levofloxacin), OR
    - IV antipseudomonal -lactam and IV aminoglycoside (gentamicin, tobramycin) plus either an IV antipneumococcal quinolone or IV macrolide
    - If documented -lactam allergy: aztreonam IV plus IV aminoglycoside plus IV antipneumococcal quinolone

Excluded Populations:

- Patients received in transfer from another acute care hospital, including another emergency department
- Patients who have no working diagnosis of pneumonia at the time of admission
- Patients receiving Comfort Measures Only
- Patients less than 18 years of age
- Patients who are compromised as defined in the data dictionary
- Patients whose initial antibiotic was administered more than 36 hours from the time of arrival
- PN patients not in the ICU
- Patients who did not receive antibiotics during hospitalization

PN-6b Initial antibiotic selection for pneumonia in immunocompetent patients non-ICU:
Immunocompetent non-intensive care unit (ICU) patients with pneumonia who receive an initial antibiotic regime during the first 24 hours that is consistent with current guidelines

Included Populations:

- All non-ICU patients, including patients transferred from long-term care facilities, on the following antibiotics:
    - -lactam IV or IM (ceftriaxone, cefotaxime, ampicillin-sulbactam) plus IV or oral macrolide (clarithromycin, azithromycin)
    - Quinolone monotherapy IV or oral levofloxacin, gatifloxacin, moxifloxacin or -lactam IV or IM plus doxycycline IV or oral

Excluded Populations:

- Patients received in transfer from another acute care hospital, including another emergency department
- Patients who have no working diagnosis of pneumonia at the time of admission
- Patients receiving Comfort Measures only
- Patients less than 18 years of age
- Patients who are compromised as defined in the data dictionary
- Patients whose initial antibiotic was administered more than 36 hours from the time of arrival
- PN patients in the ICU
- Patients who did not receive antibiotics during hospitalization

PN-7 Influenza Vaccination: Pneumonia patients age 50 years and older, hospitalized during October, November, December, January, or February with pneumonia who were screened for influenza vaccine status and were vaccinated prior to discharge, if indicated

Included Populations:

- All PN patients with physician documentation of the diagnosis of pneumonia written before or at the time of admission including patients transferred from long-term care facilities

Excluded Populations:

- Patients received in transfer from another acute care hospital, including another emergency department
- Patients who have no working diagnosis of pneumonia at the time of admission
- Patients receiving Comfort Measures Only
- Patients less than 18 years of age
- Patients who expired in the hospital
- Patients discharged to hospice care
- Patients with a principle or secondary diagnosis of 487.0 (influenza with pneumonia)
- Patients who were transferred to another short-term general hospital for inpatient care, or who were discharged/transferred to a federal hospital

Source: Brian J. Bossard, MD, founder and director, Inpatient Physician Associates, Lincoln, NE.

 © 2006 HCPRO, INC. TOOLS AND STRATEGIES FOR AN EFFECTIVE HOSPITALIST PROGRAM

| Figure | 9.3 | Hospitalist report—Pneumonia core measures initiative (cont.) |

CMS Inpatient National Quality Improvement Projects
The JCAHO ORYX Initiative/Core Measures
X Medical Center
04/01/2005 - 06/30/2005

PNEUMONIA
HOSPITALISTS REPORT

MD	PN 1[abcd] Oxygenation Assessment	PN 2[abcd] Pneumococcal Vaccination	PN 3a[a] Blood Cultures ≤ 24 hr Prior to or After Arrival	PN 3b[abc] Blood Cultures Before First Antibiotic	PN 4[abc] Adult Smoking Cessation Advice/ Counseling	PN 5[b] Antibiotic Timing (Mean)	PN 5b[abcd]** Antibiotic Timing ≤ 240 min	PN 6[a,c] Initial Antibiotic Selection	PN 6a[b] Initial Antibiotic Selection (ICU Patients)	PN 6b[b] Initial Antibiotic Selection (Non ICU Patients)	PN 7[abc] Influenza Vaccination
1	100% (2/2)	100% (2/2)	100% (2/2)	100% (2/2)	NA	312 min	0% (0/1)	100% (2/2)	NA	100% (2/2)	NA
2	100% (3/3)	100% (1/1)	100% (3/3)	100% (3/3)	50% (1/2)	528 min	50% (1/2)	100% (1/1)	100% (1/1)	NA	NA
3	100% (7/7)	75% (3/4)	71.4% (5/7)	60% (3/5)	100% (1/1)	162 min	66.7% (4/6)	NA	NA	NA	NA
4	100% (4/4)	100% (3/3)	100% (4/4)	75% (3/4)	100% (3/3)	116 min	100% (4/4)	75% (3/4)	0% (0/4)	100% (3/3)	NA
5	100% (4/4)	75% (3/4)	75% (3/4)	100% (3/3)	100% (1/1)	145 min	75% (3/4)	100% (3/3)	100% (1/1)	100% (2/2)	NA
6	100% (4/4)	100% (3/3)	100% (4/4)	100% (4/4)	100% (2/2)	148 min	100% (2/2)	100% (4/4)	NA	100% (3/3)	NA
7	100% (4/4)	100% (1/1)	100% (4/4)	75% (3/4)	100% (1/1)	92 min	100% (4/4)	75% (3/4)	100% (1/1)	75% (3/4)	NA
8	100% (7/7)	100% (4/4)	100% (7/7)	100% (7/7)	NA	144 min	100% (5/5)	75% (3/4)	NA	100% (1/1)	NA
9	100% (3/3)	100% (3/3)	100% (3/3)	66.7% (2/3)	100% (2/2)	195 min	50% (1/2)	100% (2/2)	100% (1/1)	100% (3/3)	NA
10	100% (7/7)	100% (2/2)	100% (7/7)	71.4% (5/7)	100% (2/2)	151 min	100% (6/6)	100% (6/6)	100% (3/3)	100% (3/3)	NA
11	100% (6/6)	75% (3/4)	100% (6/6)	50% (3/6)	100% (1/1)	227 min	50% (1/2)	60% (3/5)	NA	60% (3/5)	NA

Legend:

90.0 - 100% compliance	80.0 - 89.9% compliance	< 80.0% compliance	

Hospital Quality Measures Submission:
a = Centers for Medicare & Medicaid Services (CMS) - 7th Scope of Work Quality Measures
b = The Joint Commission on Accreditation of Healthcare Organizations (JCAHO) - ORYX/ Core Measures
c = Hospital Quality Alliance (HQA) Measures
d = Annual Payment Update (APU) Measures
** Studies indicate that shortening the time to first dose of antibiotics to within 4 hours of arrival is associated with improved survival rates

Improvement Plan beginning October 2003
1. The VP of Patient Care Services, and Epidemiology organized a group to finalize the Pneumonia and Influenza Standing Order Form and design a process that would support its use and facilitate vaccinations--February 2004
2. ED Medical Director addressed opportunity for ED physicians to initiate antibiotic orders while the patient is in ED--February 2004
3. Medical Staff Leadership established project champion--March 3, 2004
4. Laminates outlining clinical guidelines on PN charts--March 17, 2004
5. Medical Staff Leadership established goal of achieving ≥ 90% compliance beginning with June 2004 data--May 5, 2004
6. PN pre-printed antibiotic order revised to read "First dose STAT if not received in Emergency Department", also Pneumovax to be given before dismissal--July 2, 2004
7. Adult patient data base has been modified to include a field to collect the "pneumococcal vaccine given date"--October 13, 2004
8. Pneumovax/Influenza Standard Order implemented--October 13, 2004
9. Clinical Connection article outlining pneumonia process improvement objectives--November 11, 2004
10. Concurrent review of AMI, HF, and PN on East Progressive Care by CQI staff--December 23, 2004
11. Concurrent review of AMI, HF, and PN throughout Medical Center by CQI staff--January 17, 2005
12. Clinical Guidelines Reminders pocket booklets distributed to Medical Center staff--January 2005
13. A pop-up box has been added to the Invision Discharge Instruction sheet as a reminder to vaccinate (pneumovax/influenza) before discharge--January 2005
14. Letter to physicians concerning Initial Antibiotic Selection--April 13, 2005
15. Laminated Initial Antibiotic Selection cards to Hospitalists--June 17, 2005
16. Pharmacy will place a "Pharmacy note" in the scheduled medication section of the MAR for vaccine administration--August 5, 2005
17. Clinical Connection article reporting vaccination Milestone for pneumovax and influenza vaccinations--September 16, 2005

* Sample size = 100%

Source: Brian J. Bossard, MD, founder and director, Inpatient Physician Associates, Lincoln, NE.

CONFIDENTIAL
The content of this document is related to improving patient care.

Figure 9.4   **(Name of hospitalist service) quarterly report Identify quarter)**

Purpose: How to get your voice heard so that your critically important service receives the support it needs to continue to thrive

Strategy: Show what you are already doing and why your service is worth the investment protected time and added resources

Target Audience: Physician leaders, hospital administrators

Introduction: A positive statement highlighting last quarter's successes and plans for next quarter

- *What's new*
- *Key information (keep it brief or it will not be read)*
- *Comment on any changes in the administrative structure (do not assume this is already known)(see attached sample)*
- *A statement about the strategic focus of the hospitalist service,* (e.g., "The Hospitalist Strategic Council has identified opportunities to interact with colleagues and experts in quality improvement (QI) to address remediable challenges that our service faces. At our annual retreat we will discuss successful tactics for measuring and implementing QI initiatives.")
- *A concluding statement,* (e.g., "It is with great anticipation and enthusiasm that we look forward to the upcoming quarter, continuing to further our mission to promote high quality and efficient care, excel as educators, define the specialty of Hospital Medicine, and set the standard for inpatient care at _____ Hospital.")

Please see the enclosed documents:

- Summary of clinical staffing and clinical coverage responsibilities
- Description of new services
- Discharge volume and average daily census for hospitalist teams
- Hospitalist service report card
- Feedback from patients and primary care physicians ("customers" of service)
- Future directions

Sincerely,

| Figure | 9.4 | (Name of hospitalist service) quarterly report Identify quarter) (cont.) |

(Name of hospitalist service), **FY 2006**
Time devoted to Clinical Coverage Responsibilities

Physician	Clinical FTEs
Total, Clinical FTEs	

–Specify names, so that administrators can identify who is actually a hospitalist (versus moonlighters who do not have the same investment in the hospital).
–Indicate who has requested a reduction in clinical time and why.

Total Budgeted MD FTEs in FY06	
Actual MD FTEs in FY06	*

* Up (or down) from _____ FTE in FY05

We are actively recruiting for our open ___ FTEs. Additionally, ___ physicians on our service are scheduled to be on leave in the coming months or have requested a reduction in clinical FTEs.

Commentary on the marketplace: Current active recruitment for area hospitalist programs:

Figure 9.4 | **(Name of hospitalist service) quarterly report Identify quarter) (cont.)**

(Name of hospitalist service)
Clinical Coverage Responsibilities

This section is intended to provide information to physician leaders who might not be familiar with what the service actually does. If the service has expanded to include new primary care physician groups and/or services such as a code team, rapid response team, procedure service, or comanagement surgical model, be sure to include them in the report. These services interrupt the workday and require additional FTEs. Following the report documenting FTEs, this section of the quarterly report can serve as documentation supporting the need for additional FTEs "at a glance."

Sources of Patient Referral

Physician Clinical Coverage (weekdays)

Physician Clinical Coverage (weekends and holidays)

Medical Consultation Service (and other services covered by hospitalists)

Additional Coverage, Hospitalist Service
For example:

- 24/7 beeper coverage
- "Float" position: provides overflow, sick, and leave coverage

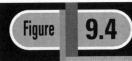

(Name of hospitalist service) quarterly report Identify quarter) (cont.)

(Name of hospitalist service)
Discharge Volume and Average Daily Census

Include comparisons with other services within general medicine and comparisons with other quarters and the same quarter in the previous year.

Data obtained from_____

The Hospitalist Report Card

The Hospitalist Report Card does not have to be all-inclusive but rather should reflect what is important to the service and the larger institution. The key is to target your effort, to perform better on two to three measures you choose so that you can demonstrate an improvement from quarter to quarter and relative to other services. Include information already being collected by the hospital such as ALOS in days, hospital readmission rate within 14 days, number of ICU transfers, and patient satisfaction data. Always indicate the source of data, which you obtain, preferably, from others so that you do not have to reinvent the wheel.

Report Card Data Commentary

This section is designed to

- *highlight the accomplishments of the service*
- *identify opportunities for improvement*
- *explain limitations of the data*
- *identify steps to be taken to make the data more actionable*

For example, if the report card shows an increase in readmission rate and a decrement in ALOS compared to a previous quarter, it is worthwhile to include possible explanations for this finding (i.e., discharging patients too soon, inadequate follow-up arranged by the discharging hospitalist, inability to book timely follow-up due to lack of PCP availability, etc.) and the steps to be taken to resolve the problem.

Patient Feedback

Include excerpts from letters sent by patients to members of the service or to the hospital to emphasize the importance of patient-centered care.

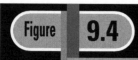

(Name of hospitalist service) quarterly report Identify quarter) (cont.)

Future Directions

This section is designed to

- *highlight cross-divisional and cross-department collaboration through rapid cycle improvements*
- *explain areas prioritized for improvement*
  - *-Rationale*
  - *-Aim*
  - *-Barriers to the plan for change*
  - *-Process and next steps*
- *showcase innovative new pilots*
  - *-Specific measurements on how the pilot is doing*

This section includes the mission statement of the service and a vision for the evolving role of the hospitalist in the next quarter.

Appendix

This section varies from quarter to quarter depending on the time of the year.

For example,

- Q1 January–March
  - Recruitment
  - Marketplace
  - New pilots

- Q2 April–June
  - PCP and other attending survey results
  - Value added summary of service in anticipation of budgetary decisions for next fiscal year

Figure 9.4 **(Name of hospitalist service) quarterly report Identify quarter) (cont.)**

- Q3 July–September
    - Annual retreat
    - Patient satisfaction/letters
    - Summary of clinical staffing and clinical coverage responsibilities

- Q4 October–December
    - Awards
    - Publications
    - Innovation

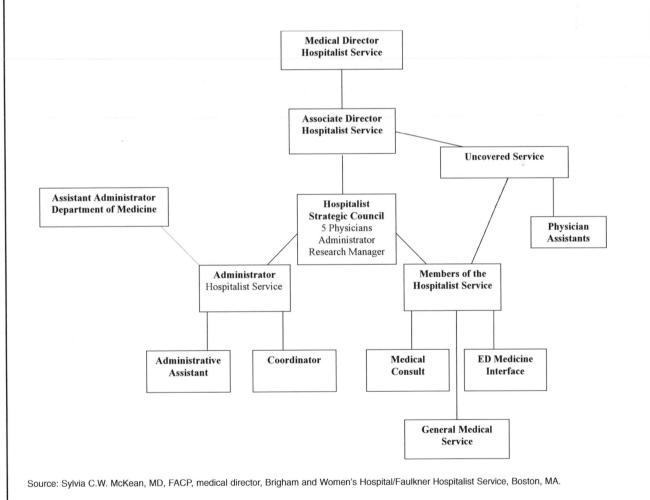

Source: Sylvia C.W. McKean, MD, FACP, medical director, Brigham and Women's Hospital/Faulkner Hospitalist Service, Boston, MA.

Considerations when linking compensation to quality measures

Before linking an agreed upon quality measure to compensation, the hospitalist service must determine

- whether the quality measure can be changed by hospitalist physicians
- the level of ease and expense involved in measuring the quality indicator
- the accuracy of measurement

For example, discharge before noon is influenced by multiple factors, some of which are beyond the hospitalist's control. This is especially true at academic centers where medical residents write discharge orders. Likewise, a hospitalist service might choose diagnosis for heart failure quality measures over diagnostic measures for acute coronary syndrome because patients with the latter diagnosis are more likely to be cared for by a cardiologist.

A hospitalist service also must decide whether individual and/or group incentives will be linked to compensation, set thresholds for quality incentives, and develop accurate provider profiling. Revenue-neutral incentives target individuals by linking compensation to individuals, but the total amount of salary support remains the same. For some hospitalist services, the only way to tie performance to any incentive is to get the hospital to set aside money that the group either receives or does not receive depending on whether specific targets are reached.

With careful planning and consensus building, hospitalist report cards should improve quality of care, reduce variability of service, provide hospitalists with benchmarks and incentives to improve performance in the six quality domains outlined at the beginning of this chapter, and enable hospital administrators to appreciate at a glance the value of a hospitalist service compared to traditional care.

References

1. The Joint Commission on Accreditation of Healthcare Organizations, Public Policy Initiatives, "Principles for the Construct of Pay-for-Performance Programs," *www.jcaho.org/about+us/public+policy+ initiatives/pay_for_performance.htm*.

2. K.G Shojania and others, "Making Healthcare Safer: A Critical Analysis of Patient Safety Practices," UCSF-Stanford Evidence-Based Practice Center/Agency for Healthcare Research and Quality, July 20, 2001. Publication 01-E058, Evidence report no. 43.

3. The Kaiser Family Foundation/Agency for Health Care Research and Quality, "Americans as Health Care Consumers: An Update on the Role of Quality Information," *www.ahrq.gov/downloads/pub/ kffsummary00.pdf*.

4. University HealthSystem Consortium, *www.uhc.edu*.

5. Institute of Medicine, Committee on Health Care in America, *Crossing the Quality Chasm: A New Health System for the 21st Century* (Washington, DC: National Academy Press, 2001): 5–6, executive summary.

6. The National Quality Forum, *www.qualityforum.org/about/home.htm*.

7. The Center for Clinical Excellence, Brigham and Women's Hospital, *www.brighamandwomens.org/ qualitycare/clinical_excellence.asp*.

8. "Brigham and Women's balanced scorecard goes hi-tech," *Data Strategy Benchmarks*, 6, no. 10 (October 2002): 145–8.

9. V.K. Sahney, "Balanced scorecard as a framework for driving performance in managed care organizations," *Managed Care Q.* 6, no. 2 (Spring 1998): 1–8.

10. George A. Steiner, *Strategic Planning: What Every Manager Must Know* (Free Press: New York, 1979).

11. D. Dranove and others, "Is More Information Better? The Effects of Report Cards on Health Care Providers," *Journal of Political Economy* 111, no. 3 (2003): 555–588.

12. Additional information on implementing quality improvement projects, specifically on rapid cycle improvement, is available on the Institute for Health Care Improvement Web site, *at www.iom.edu/CMS/3718.aspx.*

Information on pay for performance is at *www.iom.edu/CMS/3809/19805/31310.aspx.*

Additional reading

Berwick, D.M. "Continuous Improvement as an Ideal in Health Care." *New England Journal of Medicine* 320 (1989): 53–56.

Example guidelines and other quality measures available at the National Guideline Clearinghouse: *www.guideline.gov/search/searchresults.aspx?Type=3&txtSearch=venous+thromboembolism&num=20*

Kaplan, R.S., and D.P. Norton. "The Balanced Scorecard–Measures that Drive Performance." *Harvard Business Review* 70, no. 1 (Jan–Feb 1992): 71–79.

Nolan, T.W. "System Changes to Improve Patient Safety." *BMJ* 320 (March 2000): 771–772.

Preprinted orders

10

Preprinted orders

Gregory M. Susla, PharmD, FCCM

Kenneth G. Simone, DO

Handwritten physician orders for patient admissions, discharges, transfers, medications, and laboratory tests are traditionally written on generic hospital order sheets. However, during the past 25 years, preprinted orders, or ordersets, have gained popularity in the acute-care hospital setting.

The development of preprinted orders

Initially, preprinted orders were limited to surgical preoperative admission or postoperative orders and were developed for the surgeon's convenience. Surgeons' offices customized the preprinted orders for the specific type of surgery being performed. Physician- and surgery-specific ordersets grew so popular that, in many hospitals, it was not uncommon for hundreds of ordersets to exist. As a result, the preprinted orders

- lacked consistency among physicians
- were rarely updated
- contained medications not stocked by the pharmacy and not approved by the hospital's pharmacy and therapeutics committee

In addition, the past several years have seen renewed interest in preprinted ordersets as a method of standardizing therapy based on patient diagnosis (e.g., community-acquired pneumonia, acute myocardial infarction), type of physician group (e.g., orthopedic surgery), pharmacy and therapeutics committee protocols (e.g., weight-based heparin protocols), and patients' admitting location (e.g., intensive care unit admission orders, ventilator bundles). These preprinted ordersets are designed to promote standard practice while improving patient safety and outcomes.

Guidelines for use

In most hospitals today, any physician or department may request preprinted orders. However, hospitals, departments, and individual physicians should take steps to ensure patient safety and outcomes before implementing these orders:

- Department chiefs or medical directors should review and sign off on all preprinted orders likely to be used in their clinical area.

- Authors of preprinted ordersets should solicit feedback from interdisciplinary team members who are expected to use the ordersets. In addition, the clinician or committee authoring the orderset has primary responsibility for ensuring that the request moves through the approval process in a timely manner.

- The pharmacy must review all preprinted ordersets to ensure the accuracy and appropriateness of all the medications and doses included on the ordersets.

- The appropriate interdisciplinary team should review preprinted ordersets at least every three years or as clinical practice standards change.

- Each preprinted orderset should include a tracking number and a revision date.

Solutions for tracking and organizing ordersets

Finalized, preprinted orders used on general nursing units, in operating room suites, and in emergency departments are often stored in ward-based file cabinets. Unfortunately, in this type of setting, the preprinted ordersets are usually lost and rarely restocked or replaced with updated forms. Further complicating the matter, rarely is any one individual charged with keeping the ordersets in his or her clinical area up to date.

To combat the problem, many institutions are storing preprinted ordersets on ward-based computer desktops or on the hospital's intranet system. The ordersets may be placed in electronic files based on specific drugs, disease states, or physician groups.

Format and contents of ordersets

Preprinted ordersets should contain, when appropriate,

- code status
- vital signs
- diagnostic tests
- diet
- activity
- consultations
- generic drug names

Ordersets with multiple order options must include check boxes next to the options. Blank spaces (indicating dose, duration, etc.) must be filled in. All orders are considered active unless crossed out.

Other guidelines to keep in mind when creating or revising order sets include the following:

- The hospital's pharmacy and therapeutics committees' policies must be reflected on all preprinted ordersets.

- Generic drug names must be used on all preprinted ordersets, and medication allergies must be included on all preprinted ordersets containing medications.

- No statements such as "may use home medications" or "continue preop medications" should be used.

- The use of abbreviations should be minimized, no trailing zeros should be used, and drugs should be designated by metric weight rather than by number of tablets, capsules, etc.

- Nonformulary medications should not be included on preprinted ordersets.

- No orders should be printed on the backs of the order sheets. The backs may be used for supplementary information and guidelines only.

Special considerations for pain medication orders

Orders prescribing pain medications require additional considerations. Those including acetaminophen-containing pain medications should include the statement, "Total acetaminophen not to exceed 4000 mg in 24 hours"; must list the acetaminophen content of each product; and should include a non-acetaminophen-containing pain medication, such as oxycodone.

Preprinted orders with pain medications should include an agent for oral administration so that patients can be transitioned to oral therapy when appropriate. Orders for parenteral pain management should include a parenteral route other than intramuscular (IM), such as intravenous (IV) or IV patient-controlled anesthesia. Orders containing narcotic analgesics/benzodiazepines should include orders for rescue therapy (naloxone/flumazenil).

Figures 10.1–10.5 are examples of preprinted ordersets that can be used as templates to develop forms that meet the needs of individual institutions.

Figure 10.1 TNK (Tenecteplase—tPA) for myocardial infarction orders

St. Joseph Hospital
360 Broadway
Bangor, ME 04401

Preprinted Orders

Drug allergies	Patient identification

Date/time	TNK (Tenecteplase – tPA) for Myocardial Infarction Orders Page 1 of 2	Nurse's initials
	A. PRE-TNK	
	1. EKG STAT	
*	2. NTG_____ mg SL: repeat q5min x 2 prn chest pain (For total of 3 doses)	
	3. ☐ Repeat EKG (optional) if pain not relieved	
*	4. STAT labs:	
	a. ☐ Blood type (ABO/Rh) and Antibody Screen (for possible blood transfusion)	
	b. ☐ X-match_____ units (for probable blood transfusion)	
	c. ☐ CBC/BMP (Basic Metabolic Panel), Mg level	
	d. ☐ PT, PTT, Fibrinogen	
	e. ☐ CIS protocol	
	5. Portable CXR (reason: chest pain). May be done after TNK started.	
	6. Start 3 IV lines (at least one 18g or larger). Cap as Saline Locks with routine flushes if not needed.	
	7. BABY ASA 324 mg PO (81 mg X 4 tabs) – Give STAT and have patient chew tablets	
	B. TNK (Tenecteplase)	
	1. Reconstitute TNK with sterile water	
	2. Check one of the following dosage options:	

Patient Weight (kg)	TNKase (mg)	mL of reconstituted TNKase
☐ <60 (kg)	30 mg IV	6
☐ ≥60 to <70	35 mg IV	7
☐ ≥70 to <80	40 mg IV	8
☐ ≥80 to <90	45 mg IV	9
☐ ≥90	50 mg IV	10

Date/time		Nurse's initials
*	**C. Heparin**	
	1. Heparin 60 units/kg IV bolus (not to exceed 4,000 units). Give within 1 hour of starting TNK. (Bolus = _____ units)	

	2. Mix IV Heparin drip in the following concentration:
	   ____ 25,000 units/500 ml D5W (Standard)
	   ____ 25,000 units/250 ml D5W	

	3. Start IV Heparin infusion at 12 units/kg/hr (not to exceed 1,000 units/hr) (Rate = _____ units.hr)	
*	**D. ADJUNCTIVE THERAPY OPTIONS: CHECK DESIRED MEDICATIONS**	
	☐ Metoprolol 5 mg IV q5min x 3 doses, then Metoprolol 50 mg PO q6h (Start 15 min after last IV dose). Hold Metoprolol if systolic BP less than 100 or pulse less than 60.	
	☐ IV Nitroglycerine (100 mg/250 ml D5W = 400 mcg/ml). Start infusion at 0.5 mcg/kg/min. Titrate for relief of chest pain. Maintain systolic BP greater than 100.	
	☐ Famotidine (Pepcid) 20 mg PO bid. Discontinue when off Heparin.	
	☐ Enalapril (Vasotec) _____ mg PO q12hrs.	
	☐ Captopril (Capoten) _____ mg PO q8hrs.	

Use ballpoint pen only
*Physician required to write in a choice or preference

*Source: **St. Joseph Hospital**, 360 Broadway, Bangor, ME*

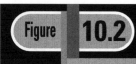

Inpatient medical service physician's orders

St. Joseph Hospital
360 Broadway
Bangor, ME 04401

Preprinted Orders

Drug allergies

Patient identification

Date/time	INPATIENT MEDICAL SERVICE PHYSICIAN'S ORDERS — Page 1 of 2	Nurse's initials
	Admit to: Location:	
	Diagnosis:	
	DNR Status:	
	Telemetry: ☐ yes ☐ no	
	Allergies: ☐ none known ☐ list all known:	
	Case management: ☐ yes ☐ no	
	Social Services: ☐ yes ☐ no	
	Vital Signs: ☐ routine ☐ every shift ☐ other	
	Weight: ☐ on admission ☐ daily ☐ other	
	Intake & Output: ☐ yes ☐ no	
	☐ Foley Catheter ☐ Condom Catheter ☐ other	
	Blood Glucose Monitoring: ☐ qid-ac and hs ☐ bid ac breakfast & supper ☐ other	
	Diet: ☐ NPO ☐ NPO except ice chips ☐ NPO except sips of water and meds	
	☐ Cardiac ☐ Renal ☐ 2 gm Sodium	
	☐ Clear liquids ☐ Full liquids ☐ Pureed	
	☐ Mechanical soft ☐ Low residue ☐ Other	
	☐ Advance as Tolerated	
	☐ Diabetic Diet: ☐ No Concentrated Sweets	
	☐ Calories (Specify) _____ ADA	
	☐ Fluid restriction _____ ml/Day	
	Activity: ☐ AD LIB ☐ With Assist ☐ Bed Rest	
	☐ Bedside Commode ☐ With Assist ☐ Bed to Chair	
	☐ Advance as tolerated ☐ Cardiac steps by nurse protocol	
	Therapy:	
	☐ Cardiac Rehab Consult	
	☐ Physical Therapy: Evaluate and Treat	
	☐ Occupational Therapy: Evaluate and Treat	
	☐ Speech Therapy: Evaluate and Treat	
	☐ Swallowing Evaluation	
	☐ Modified Barium Swallow	
	IV: ☐ Fluid_____ Rate:_____ Duration:_____	
	☐ Saline Lock_____	
	Labs: ☐ Cardiac Injury Series ☐ TSH ☐ HGBA$_1$C	
	Profiles: ☐ CBC ☐ BMP ☐ CMP ☐ Liver ☐ Coag ☐ Lipid	
	☐ Other_____	
	☐ Blood culture X 2_____	
	☐ Stool for occult blood _____ X_____	

Use ballpoint pen only
*Physician required to write in a choice or preference

   © 2006 HCPRO, INC.   **TOOLS AND STRATEGIES FOR AN EFFECTIVE HOSPITALIST PROGRAM**

Figure **10.2**   Inpatient medical service physician's orders (cont.)

Date/ time	INPATIENT MEDICAL SERVICE PHYSICIAN'S ORDERS — Page 2 of 2	Nurse's initials
	X-Ray: ☐ Chest – Portable Indication:	
	☐ Chest – PA & LAT Indication:	
	☐ ABD Series Indication:	
	☐ CT of With contrast	
	Without contrast	
	Indication:	
	Other Indication:	
	Cardiac Studies: ☐ EKG ☐ Echocardiogram	
	Treadmill: ☐ Standard	
	☐ With Sestamibi	
	☐ Persantine Sestamibi	
	☐ Dobutamine echocardiogram	
	☐ RVG	
	☐ Other	
	Protocols:	
	☐ Potassium: ☐ PO ☐ IV See separate order sheet	
	☐ Magnesium: ☐ PO ☐ IV See separate order sheet	
	☐ Insulin: See separate order sheet	
	☐ Heparin: IV, Weight-based ☐ See separate order sheet	
	☐ Joint Practice: See separate order sheet	
	☐ Metered Dose Inhaler: See separate order sheet	
	☐ Other:	
	Medications:	
	☐ Tylenol mg po/pr q4h prn: Pain or temperature over	
	☐ Maalox ml po q4h prn: Indigestion	
	☐ Restoril mg po hs prn: Sleep	
	☐ Ambien mg po hs prn: Sleep	
	☐ Benadryl mg po hs prn: Sleep	
	☐ Laxative of choice:	
	Nausea:	
	☐ Benadryl mg IV q4h prn	
	☐ Phenergan mg pr/po/IM/IV q4h prn	
	☐ Reglan 10 mg po/IV q6h prn	
	☐ Compazine mg po/IV q6h prn	
	☐ Zofran mg po/IV q6h prn	
	☐ O$_2$ at L/MIN by nasal cnnula	
	☐ Maximum O$_2$ sat at % adjust q h	
	DVT Prophylaxis	
	☐ Lovenox 30 mg sq q12h	
	☐ Heparin 5000 units sq q12h	
	☐ Sequential stockings	
	Other Medications:	
	1)	
	2)	
	3)	
	4)	
	5)	
	6)	
	Physician Signature: Date	

Use ballpoint pen only
*Physician required to write in a choice or preference
Source: St. Joseph Hospital, 360 Broadway, Bangor, ME

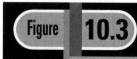

Observation orders—Congestive heart failure

St. Joseph Hospital
360 Broadway
Bangor, ME 04401

Preprinted Orders

Drug allergies	Patient identification

Date/ time	OBSERVATION ORDERS — CHF Page 1 of 1	Nurse's initials
	OBSERVATION to CPCU with Telemetry service of Dr. _____	
	Dx: **CHF**	
	Vital Signs q shift	
	PULSE OX in AM	
	Activity as tolerated	
	Nursing: I & O q shift	
	Weigh patient q AM	
	Diet: Cardiac Prudent Low Sodium	
	Fluid Restriction: 1-1.5L / 2-2.5L/day	
	Saline Lock	
	Labs in AM: BMP, Mg	
	EKG — if not done in ED	
	CXR – PA / LAT or PCXR in AM if not done in ED	
	☐ O$_2$:	
	Meds / Protocols:	
	Physician signature:_____ Date:_____	

Use ballpoint pen only
***Physician required to write in a choice or preference**

*Source: **St. Joseph Hospital**, 360 Broadway, Bangor, ME*

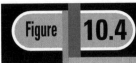

Observation orders—Chest pain

St. Joseph Hospital

360 Broadway
Bangor, ME 04401

Preprinted Orders

Drug allergies	Patient identification

Date/ time	OBSERVATION ORDERS — CHEST PAIN Page 1 of 1	Nurse's initials
	OBSERVATION to CPCU with Telemetry service of Dr. _____	
	Dx: **CHEST PAIN**	
	Vital Signs q shift	
	Activity: Out of bed as tolerated after a negative Troponin Series	
	Nursing: I & O q shift	
	Weigh patient on admission	
	Diet: Cardiac Prudent Low Sodium	
	Saline Lock	
	Labs: **TROPONIN SERIES**	
	Cholesterol Profile	
	BMP in AM	
	EKG in AM	
	Meds: ASA Enteric Coated 325 mg q daily	
	Nitro 0.4 mg sl q 5min x3 prn	
	Morphine Sulfate 2–4 mg IV q 10min prn	
	O_2 – 2l nc prn CP or SOB	
	Other Meds / Protocol:	
	Testing:	
	Physician signature: Date: _____	

Use ballpoint pen only
*Physician required to write in a choice or preference

*Source: **St. Joseph Hospital**, 360 Broadway, Bangor, ME*

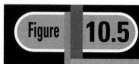

Observation orders—Asthma

St. Joseph Hospital
360 Broadway
Bangor, ME 04401

Preprinted Orders

Drug allergies	Patient identification

Date/time	OBSERVATION ORDERS — ASTHMA Page 1 of 1	Nurse's initials
	OBSERVATION to CPCU with Telemetry service of Dr. _____	
	Dx: ASTHMA	
	Vital Signs q shift	
	Activity: Ad Lib	
	Nursing: I & O q shift	
	PULSE OX in AM	
	Diet:	
	Saline Lock	
	Labs: ABG prn	
	CBC	
	☐ O_2:	
	Meds: **NEBS:** Albuterol 2.5 / Atrovent 0.5 q2hr, q4hr with	
	Albuterol 2.5 q1hr prn.	
	D/C Orders:	
	Steroids:	
	Physician signature: _____ Date: _____	

Use ballpoint pen only
*Physician required to write in a choice or preference

Source: **St. Joseph Hospital,** *360 Broadway, Bangor, ME*

 © 2006 HCPro, Inc. **TOOLS AND STRATEGIES FOR AN EFFECTIVE HOSPITALIST PROGRAM**

Coding and compliance for the inpatient physician

11

Coding and compliance for the inpatient physician

Charleen A. Porter, BA, MA, CPC

Current coding environment

The current financial atmosphere in medicine is one of increasing auditing and review. Physicians are being challenged to produce more and document more, yet are rewarded with decreasing reimbursement. As a result, it is extremely important for hospitalists to understand coding, make the right coding choices, and support their choices with adequate documentation.

Hospitalists also must understand that putting appropriate information into the patient record serves multiple purposes, as follows:

- First, the record should contain a thorough description of the patient's condition and a complete listing of services provided to give other physicians and caregivers a clear picture of the patient's condition and status.

- Second, the information in the patient record will determine whether the physician keeps what the insurer has paid out for the services rendered, should the physician be the target of an audit. Documentation of the hospitalist's thinking process helps support the medical necessity of the services provided or ordered.

- Third, the patient's record supports the hospitalist's thinking process and choice of treatments and management options, should he or she be questioned in court regarding the patient's outcome.

- Fourth, pay for performance is on the horizon. The documentation of certain protocols or best practices will determine whether the hospitalist will receive reimbursement incentives under a pay-for-performance model.

Increased auditing activity

Historically, much of the attention surrounding auditing activity focused on the Centers for Medicare & Medicaid Services' (CMS) strategies and initiatives, and commercial insurers were willing to let the government do the legwork. However, commercial insurers are beginning to move forward with their own auditing initiatives, due in large part to the fact that Medicare demonstrated how examining documentation can lead to huge monetary refunds to the auditor.

When shopping for an insurer, hospitals, inpatient medicine programs, and hospitalists should understand that not all auditors are created equal. Remember, the purpose is to recover funds. Physicians should not hesitate to contact a healthcare consultant and ask for a second opinion on whether the documentation supports the level of service billed. Likewise, they should not hesitate to challenge an insurer when they are sure the documentation and medical necessity for a service supports the level of care in question. All insurers have avenues for appeal.

Medicare's latest effort in the realm of auditing involves recovery audit contractors (RAC). For more information on this initiative, refer to the Helpful Resources section at the end of this chapter.

Progressive corrective action

Progressive corrective action is a process that CMS contractors are instructed to use to educate physicians when a medical review uncovers a problem with the physician's documentation. It entails a series of efforts the contractor should make to educate the physician when the error discovered does not constitute fraud. For more information on progressive corrective action, see the Helpful resources section at the end of this chapter.

Pay for performance

At press time, the government had not yet released a finalized, official pay-for-performance model. However, as noted, there is little doubt that this initiative is on the horizon. To find out more about pay for performance, refer to the Web sites listed in the Helpful resources section at the end of this chapter.

Evaluation and management documentation guidelines

The CMS released evaluation and management (E/M) documentation guidelines in late 1994 and published an expanded and revised set of the guidelines in 1997. Although the American Medical Association (AMA) and the Health Care Financing Administration (now CMS) initially developed the guidelines, nearly all insurers now follow some form of the guidelines when auditing or reviewing medical documentation. Hospitalists should note that because the E/M documentation guidelines have been available for more than ten years, tolerance for ignorance of the guidelines has expired.

Commonly referred to as the 1995 and 1997 E/M guidelines, they can be found on the CMS Web site, which is referenced at the end of this chapter.

Challenges to determining the level of service

Answers to the following questions help determine the level of service that hospitalists have provided to a patient:

- How can I better distinguish between a level two and level three admission?
- How can I better distinguish between a level two and level three subsequent inpatient visit?
- How can I more accurately choose between a level three, four, or five consultation?
- What must I put on paper to justify my critical care time?

Hospitalists often remember *types* of problems. They may not remember how many bullet points are needed for a particular level of service under the 1997 guidelines. They may not even remember a particular patient's name. However, ask a hospitalist, "Do you recall the patient with Parkinson's and chronic obstructive pulmonary disease (COPD) who you had to intubate?" and he or she will respond with full details of the patient's condition, as well as a description of the inpatient stay and prognosis.

For this reason, base the approach to choosing levels of service on the number of problems and problem types to aid the hospitalist in choosing a code. It does not negate the need to document to the level required for the level of service chosen. Documentation for the sake of documentation is not helpful. Instruct hospitalists to document what the problems are, their severity, what was examined, their thinking process and assessment, and the treatment(s) or management options they selected for the patient.

Medical necessity

The first question an insurer will ask is, "Is this level of service necessary to address the patient's problem(s)?" If the answer is "No," then even copious amounts of documentation will not support the medical necessity of the service, even though the documentation requirements for the level of service chosen are met.

The difference between level two and level three admission services

Both level two and level three admission services must meet all three key criteria for history, exam, and medical decision-making. Both levels of service require a comprehensive history and exam. The level two service requires medical decision-making of moderate complexity. The level three service requires medical decision-making of high complexity.

Medical decision-making refers to the complexity of establishing a diagnosis or selecting a management option(s). Complexity is affected by

- the number of diagnoses/the number of management options that must be considered, which in turn are based on the number and types of problems the physician will address during the encounter

- the amount and complexity of medical records, diagnostic tests, and other information that must be gathered, reviewed, and analyzed

- the risk of significant complications, morbidity/mortality, and comorbidities associated with the patient's problems, diagnostic procedures, and any other management options being considered

Moderate complexity medical decision-making

In a case of moderate complexity, the patient has multiple problems. There is a moderate amount of data to be ordered/reviewed. The risk to the patient is moderate, and he or she may have one or more chronic illnesses with mild exacerbation, progression, or side effects of treatment.

The patient may present with an undiagnosed new problem with an uncertain prognosis or an acute illness with systemic symptoms. Management options may include minor surgery/endoscopy without additional risk factors, elective major surgery, therapeutic nuclear medicine, and intravenous fluids with additives. This patient has numerous problems that need management, and he or she may be very uncomfortable, but he or she is not at imminent risk of death.

High-complexity medical decision-making

In a high-complexity case, the patient has extensive problems. The amount of data to be ordered or reviewed is extensive. The risk to the patient is high, and he or she may have one or more chronic illnesses with a severe exacerbation or progression of the disease, or side effects of treatment.

The patient may present with acute or chronic illnesses or injuries that pose a threat to life or bodily function. He or she may have experienced an abrupt change in neurologic status. Examples might include acute myocardial infarction, pulmonary embolus, and severe respiratory distress. Management options might include major surgery with identified risk factors, emergency major surgery, parenteral controlled substances, and decision not to resuscitate or to deescalate care due to poor prognosis. This patient numerous severe problems that need management and that at any time may degrade and require critical-care services.

Table 11.1 demonstrates high-complexity versus moderate-complexity decision-making.

Additional examples might include any type of life support, managing a ventilator or continuous positive airway pressure (CPAP) mask for respiratory failure, or managing vasopressors to support blood pressure for patients in shock.

Both services must meet *all three* key criteria for history, exam, and medical decision-making. Both services require a comprehensive history and exam. The level two service requires medical decision-making of moderate complexity. The level three service requires medical decision-making of high complexity.

Table 11.1			Level 2 and level 3 admission comparison			

History	Exam	Problem type	Amount of data to be ordered/ reviewed	Risk of complications and/or morbidity or mortality	Type of decision making	Level of service
Comprehensive	Comprehensive	Multiple	Moderate	Moderate	Moderate complexity	Level Two 99222
Comprehensive	Comprehensive	Extensive	Extensive	High	High complexity	Level Three 99223

Tables 11.2–11.4 demonstrate medical decision-making criteria.

Because the patient is being admitted as an inpatient, the majority of problems will likely fall into the moderate- to high-complexity category. Admission services do not distinguish between new or established patients. If the physician has managed the patient during a previous inpatient stay, the patient's problems may be considered established problems.

A level two admission will address more than one problem. It may address one worsening problem along with managing a second stable problem. For example, the patient may be admitted with a COPD or heart failure exacerbation, as well as stable diabetes.

Clinical examples

Note: The clinical examples that follow were chosen in an effort to illustrate the differences between moderate complexity, high complexity, and critical care services. They were neither approved nor endorsed by the AMA, CMS, or any other official entity. Additional clinical examples may be found in Appendix C of the *Current Procedural Terminology (CPT)* book published by the AMA.

Our patient is over 65; has mild dementia, arthritis, and a pacemaker; is diabetic; and has COPD. We will use this patient to describe presentations that we believe would be examples of a level two admis-

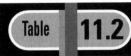

Table 11.2	**Problem types associated with low-, moderate-, and high-complexity medical decision-making**

Problem type
Established problem worsening/failing to change as expected
New problem; no additional workup planned
New problem; additional workup planned

sion, a level three admission, and a critical care service.

99222—Level two admission example

The patient presents with fever, chills, cough, dyspnea, and dyspnea on exertion. Physical exam is consistent with diffuse expiratory wheezes and rales at the right lung base. Chest x-ray is consistent with hyperexpanded lung fields consistent with COPD and right lower lobe infiltrate. The ABG reveals a p02 of 70 on 3 liters of oxygen, pH 7.45, pC02of 35, and a bicarbonate of 24. The patient is diagnosed with right lower lobe pneumonia (possible aspiration) and COPD exacerbation. She is started on nasal cannula oxygen, antibiotics, bronchodilators, and steroids. She also has her diabetes regimen adjusted because her diabetes is out of control from her pre-hospitalization regimen.

A level three admission may have the patient presenting with two established problems that are worsening, or presenting with a new problem that needs workup as well as a combination of other stable or worsening problems. There are numerous combinations of problems that fit into this category. The point is that the presenting problems are numerous and require inpatient status and a high level of physician attention to manage.

99223—Level three admission example

The patient presents with fever, chills, cough, dyspnea, and dyspnea on exertion. Physical exam is consistent with diffuse expiratory wheezes and rales at the right lung base. Chest x-ray is consistent with hyperexpanded lung fields consistent with COPD and right lower lobe infiltrate. The patient demonstrates severe hypoxemia requiring high flow oxygen therapy (50% 02). The ABG reveals a p02 of 70 on 50% oxygen, pH 7.35, pC02of 45, and a bicarbonate of 24. The pacemaker is functioning, but the patient has developed rapid atrial fibrillation requiring acute therapy.

Dementia has evolved into depression of consciousness, and the patient's diabetes is not controlled. The patient is diagnosed with right lower lobe pneumonia (possible aspiration) and COPD exacerbation. She is started on oxygen, antibiotics, bronchodilators, and steroids. She also has her diabetes regimen adjusted due to the fact that her diabetes is out of control from her pre-hospitalization regimen.

Table 11.3	Data to be ordered and/or reviewed

Review and/or order of tests in CPT Radiology Section (nuclear medicine and all imaging except echocardiography and cardiac catheter) (CPT 70000 codes)
Review and/or order of clinical lab tests (CPT 80000 codes)
Review and/or order of tests in CPT Medicine Section (EEG, EKG, echocardiography, cardiac cathether, noninvasive vascular studies, pulmonary function studies) (CPT 90000 codes)
Discussion of test results with performing physician
Independent review of image, tracing, or specimen
Decision to obtain old records and/or obtain history from someone other than the patient
Review and summarization of old records and/or history obtained from someone other than the patient

The patient's condition may require tests from multiple sections of the CPT book, as well as a review of old records. Generally, the more complex the patient's case, the more data that will need to be gathered either by ordering testing or by thoroughly reviewing the patient's past medical experiences. When the patient's medical history is reviewed, the review and summary should be documented.

The level two patient's risk will fall into the moderate risk category. The level three patient's risk will fall into the high-risk category. The difference between level two problems and level three problems is not necessarily the number of problems but the severity of the problems. The difference between a mild exacerbation and a severe exacerbation is a judgment call made by the physician. Level three admission services will apply to the most challenging patients who do not meet the critical care requirements. If the physician feels that the patient's problems demand high complexity medical decision-making, he or she should be prepared to document this clearly in the medical record. If the critical care requirements are met, then critical care services should be billed rather than level three inpatient admission services.

Table 11.4	Moderate-risk vs. high-risk examples

Level of risk	Presenting problems	Diagnostic procedures ordered	Management options
Moderate	• One or more chronic illnesses with mild exacerbation or progression, or side effect of treatment • Two or more stable chronic illnesses • Undiagnosed new problem with uncertain prognosis (e.g., lump in breast) • Acute illness with systemic symptoms (e.g., pnuemonitis, colitis, pyelonephritis) • Acute complicated injury (e.g., head injury with brief loss of consciousness)	• Physiologic tests under stress (e.g., cardiac stress test, fetal contraction stress test) • Diagnostic endoscopies with no identified risk factors • Deep needle or incisional biopsy • Cardiovascular imaging studies with contrast and no identified risk factors (e.g., arteriogram, cardiac catheterization) • Obtain fluid from body cavity (e.g., lumbar puncture, culdocentesis)	• Minor surgery with identified risk factors • Elective major surgery (open, percutaneous, or endoscopic) • Prescription drug management • Therapeutic nuclear medicine • IV fluids with additives • Closed treatment of fracture or dislocation without manipulation
High	• One or more chronic illnesses with severe exacerbation or progression or side effect of treatment • Acute or chronic illnesses or injuries that may pose a threat to life or bodily function (e.g., multiple trauma, acute myocardial infarction, pulmonary embolus, severe respiratory distress, progressive severe rheumatoid arthritis, psychiatric illness with potential threat to self or others, peritonitis, acute renal failure) • Abrupt change in neurologic status (e.g., sensory loss, seizure)	• Cardiovascular imaging studies with contrast with identified risk factors • Cardiac electrophysiological tests • Diagnostic endoscopies with identified risk factors • Discography	• Elective major surgery (open, percutaneous, or endoscopic) • Emergency major surgery (open, percutaneous, or endoscopic) • Parenteral controlled substances • Drug therapy requiring intensive monitoring for toxicity • Decision not to resuscitate or to deescalate care because of poor prognosis

| Table 11.5 | Level 2 and level 3 subsequent hospital visit comparison |

History	Exam	Problem type	Amount of data to be ordered/ reviewed	Risk of complications and/or morbidity or mortality	Type of decision making	Level of service
Expanded Problem Focused	Expanded Problem Focused	Multiple	Moderate	Moderate	Moderate complexity	Level Two 99232
Detailed	Detailed	Extensive	Extensive	High	High complexity	Level Three 99233

Differences between a level two and level three subsequent hospital visit

Subsequent hospital visits require *two of three* key components of history, exam, and medical decision-making. Current communication from CMS indicates that when a level three subsequent visit is chosen, high complexity medical decision-making must be demonstrated.

(See Tables 11.2–11.4 for medical decision-making criteria. The requirements for supporting high complexity medical decision-making are the same regardless of the type of service being considered.)

CPT describes the level two subsequent hospital visit (99232) as typically consisting of "25 minutes at the bedside and on the patient's hospital floor or unit." The level three subsequent hospital visit (99233) typically consists of "35 minutes at the bedside and on the patient's hospital floor or unit." If more than 50% of the time spent face to face with the patient is consumed by counseling the patient or patient and family regarding the patient's management, prognosis, etc., or in coordination of care, the service may be billed using time as the key component. The time spent in counseling or coordination of care activities should be documented in the record.

There are numerous clinical examples listed for 99232 and 99233 in Appendix C of the CPT book.

Table 11.6 Differences between level three, four, and five consultations

History	Exam	Problem type	Amount of data to be ordered/ reviewed	Risk of complications and/or morbidity or mortality	Type of decision making	Level of service
Detailed	Detailed	Limited	Limited	Low	Low complexity	Level three 99253
Comprehensive	Comprehensive	Multiple	Moderate	Moderate	Moderate complexity	Level four 99254
Comprehensive	Comprehensive	Extensive	Extensive	High	High complexity	Level five 99255

Differences between level three, four, and five consultations

All *three* key criteria of history, exam, and medical decision-making must be met when using these codes.

Level three problems will require less data gathering and less complex medical decision-making than level four and five services. Generally, a level three problem will be a problem that may be getting worse but for which the management options are clear or more easily defined. A level three problem may also be a new problem that does not require additional workup beyond a review of the patient's past medical experiences. The patient's risk associated with the management options chosen would be low.

The difference between the level four and level five consultations would actually be very similar to the difference between the level two and three inpatient admission. The difference may not necessarily be the number of problems but the severity of problems. The differences may lie in the amount of data that must be gathered and the risk to the patient. If the physician feels the patient falls into the high complexity category, he or she must be prepared to provide documentation sufficient to support high complexity medical decision-making and determination that there is heightened risk to the patient.

Table 11.7 gives examples of low-, moderate-, and high-risk problems.

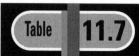

| | Low-, moderate-, and high-risk examples |

Level of risk	Presenting problems	Diagnostic procedures ordered	Management options
Low	• Two or more self-limited or minor problems • One stable chronic illness (e.g., well-controlled hypertension or noninsulin dependent diabetes, cataract, BPH) • Acute uncomplicated illness or injury (e.g., cystitis, simple sprain, allergic rhinitis)	• Physiologic tests not under stress (e.g., pulmonary function tests) • Noncardiovascular imaging studies with contrast (e.g., barium enema) • Superficial needle biopsies • Clinical lab tests requiring arterial puncture • Skin biopsies	• Over the counter drugs • Minor surgery with no identified risk factors • Physical therapy • Occupational therapy • IV fluids without additives
Moderate	• One or more chronic illnesses with mild exacerbation or progression, or side effect of treatment • Two or more stable chronic illnesses • Undiagnosed new problem with uncertain prognosis (e.g., lump in breast) • Acute illness with systemic symptoms (e.g., pnuemonitis, colitis, pyelonephritis) • Acute complicated injury (e.g., head injury with brief loss of consciousness)	• Physiologic tests under stress (e.g., cardiac stress test, fetal contraction stress test) • Diagnostic endoscopies with no identified risk factors • Deep needle or incisional biopsy • Cardiovascular imaging studies with contrast and no identified risk factors (e.g., arteriogram, cardiac catheterization) • Obtain fluid from body cavity (e.g., lumbar puncture, culdocentesis)	• Minor surgery with identified risk factors • Elective major surgery (open percutaneous, or endoscopic) • Prescription drug management • Therapeutic nuclear medicine • IV fluids with additives • Closed treatment of fracture or dislocation without manipulation
High	• One or more chronic illnesses with severe exacerbation or progression or side effect of treatment • Acute or chronic illnesses or injuries that may pose a threat to life or bodily function (e.g., multiple trauma, acute MI, pulmonary embolus, severe respiratory distress, progressive severe rheumatoid arthritis, psychiatric illness with potential threat to self or others, peritonitis, acute renal failure) • Abrupt change in neurologic status (e.g., sensory loss, seizure)	• Cardiovascular imaging studies with contrast with identified risk factors • Cardiac electrophysiological tests • Diagnostic endoscopies with identified risk factors • Discography	• Elective major surgery (open percutaneous, or endoscopic) • Emergency major surgery (open, percutaneous, or endoscopic) • Parenteral controlled substances • Drug therapy requiring intensive monitoring for toxicity • Decision not to resuscitate or to deescalate care because of poor prognosis

Use of consultation codes

In 2006, CMS made some clarifications to its consultation services policy. Among them are the following:

- A consultation service may be provided by a physician or qualified nurse practitioner (NPP)

- A request for a consultation and the need for consultation shall be documented by the consultant in the patient's medical record and included in the requesting physician's or qualified NPP's plan of care in the patient's medical record

- A consultation service allows a physician, qualified NPP, or other appropriate source to ask another physician or qualified NPP for advice or an opinion, recommendation, suggestion, or direction, etc., in evaluating or treating a patient because that physician has expertise in a specific medical area beyond the requesting professional's knowledge

- A consultation shall not be performed as a split/shared E/M visit

Transfers of care: A transfer of care occurs when a physician or qualified NPP requests that another physician or qualified NPP take over the responsibility for managing the patient's complete care for the condition and does not expect to continue treating the patient for that condition.

When such a transfer is arranged, the requesting physician or qualified NPP is not asking for an opinion or advice about personally treating the patient and does not expect to continue treating the patient for the condition. The receiving physician or qualified NPP shall document this transfer of the patient's care to his or her service in the patient's medical record or plan of care.

In a transfer of care, the receiving physician or qualified NPP would report the appropriate new or established patient visit code according to the place of service and level of service performed and shall not report a consultation service.

If the family physician follows the inpatient but asks the inpatient physician to manage the patient's diabetes or COPD, this would be considered a transfer of care for that problem. As a result, the inpatient physician would not bill a consultation code for the first visit but would bill a subsequent hospital visit code instead.

If the family physician does not follow the patient in the inpatient setting and requests that his or her patient be admitted by the inpatient service, the physician providing the initial service to the patient as an inpatient would bill the appropriate level of admission code.

In the hospital setting, the consulting physician or qualified NPP shall use the appropriate Initial Inpatient Consultation codes (99251—99255). The Initial Inpatient Consultation may be reported only once per consultant per patient per facility admission.

Preoperative clearance: Preoperative consultations are payable for new or established patients when they are performed by any physician or qualified NPP at the request of a surgeon, as long as all of the requirements for performing and reporting the consultation codes are met and the service is medically necessary and not routine screening.

This information may be found at 30.6.10 in Chapter 12 of the *Medicare Claims Processing Manual* or in Transmittal 788, dated December 20, 2005.

Use of a consultation code indicates that the physician has been asked to consult on a *specific* aspect of the patient's condition. The request must be documented in the patient's medical record. Either the referring or the receiving physician may document the request. The consulting physician may either only consult or both consult and treat the patient. The consulting physician's opinion must be documented and shared with the referring physician. If both physicians are using a shared record as in an inpatient setting, it is not necessary for the consulting physician to send the referring physician a separate document to support the consultant's findings.

For more complete details on the E/M documentation guidelines and documenting levels of service, please refer to *The Hospitalist Program Management Guide,* published by HCPro, Inc., or to the CMS Web site for the complete E/M documentation guidelines.

Critical care services

Use of critical care in cases that are not medical emergencies: Critical care includes the care of critically ill and unstable patients who require constant physician attention, regardless of whether the patient is in the course of a medical emergency. It involves decision-making of high complexity to assess, manipulate, and support circulatory, respiratory, central nervous, metabolic, or other vital system function to prevent or treat single or multiple vital organ systems failure. It often also requires extensive interpretation of multiple databases and the application of advanced technology to manage the critically ill patient.

Critical care is usually, but not always, given in a critical care area such as the coronary care unit, intensive care unit, respiratory care unit, or emergency department. Services for a patient who is not critically ill and unstable but who happens to be in a critical care, intensive care, or other specialized care unit are reported using hospital care codes (99231–99233) or hospital consultation codes (99251–99263).

The duration of critical care to be reported is the time the physician spent working on the critical care patient's case, whether the physician spent that time at the immediate bedside or elsewhere on the floor (but was immediately available to the patient). See CPT for the complete guidelines for Critical Care Services.

Critical care example

The patient presents with fever, chills, cough, dyspnea, and dyspnea on exertion. The physical exam is consistent with diffuse expiratory wheezes and rales at the right lung base. Chest x-ray is consistent with hyperexpanded lung fields consistent with COPD and right lower lobe infiltrate. The patient demonstrates evidence of acute and frank respiratory failure. Bipap therapy is started in the hopes of avoiding the need for intubation and mechanical ventilation. The patient is admitted to the ICU for an aggressive respiratory regimen, high-flow oxygen, and monitoring due to high risk of requiring mechanical ventilation. The ABG reveals a p02 of 65 on 100% oxygen, pH 7.25, pC02of 60, and a bicarbonate of 30. The pacemaker is functioning, but the patient has developed rapid atrial fibrillation requiring acute therapy. Dementia has evolved into depression of consciousness and the patient's diabetes is not controlled. The patient is diagnosed with right lower lobe pneumonia (possible aspiration) and COPD exacerbation. She is started on oxygen, IV antibiotics, bronchodilators, and steroids. She also has her diabetes regimen adjusted due to the fact that her diabetes was out of control from her pre-hospitalization regimen.

Many physicians have trouble defining critical care services. Physician groups who provide critical care must communicate with each other to develop broad parameters defining critical care services. These parameters should be used to guide the group in making similar decisions when choosing critical care codes.

Critical care services should not be chosen when one physician is covering for another and a non-critically ill but complex patient consumes a lot of face-to-face time. This service should be billed using the appropriate level for a subsequent hospital visit plus a prolonged service code, if the time exceeds the time included in the chosen code by 30 or more minutes.

Approach your Medicare carrier's medical director for review of and feedback on the broad parameters you have outlined. Your carrier medical director should help you define and clarify critical care services and their documentation.

In many states, the primary reason critical care services are denied or downcoded is the lack of documentation to support the time spent performing critical care services. By CPT definition, critical care services are time-based codes. If a physician does not clearly document the amount of time spent providing critical care services, contractors will not give credit for the critical care services.

For other sources of information on critical care services, see the Helpful resources section at the end of this chapter.

CPT changes for 2006

Two series of CPT codes were eliminated in 2006. They are Follow-Up Inpatient Consultations, CPT codes 99261–99263, and Confirmatory Consultations, CPT codes 99271–99275. Both sets of codes were eliminated due to the confusion surrounding their use.

Follow-up Inpatient Consultation codes were to be used when the consultation could not be completed or a definitive assessment could not be made at the initial encounter. This series of codes was also used when the attending physician requested a subsequent consultative visit. Physicians are now instructed to use the subsequent hospital visit codes for these types of service. If the physician is requested to consult on a different aspect of the patient's condition, use of an inpatient consultation code would be appropriate.

Confirmatory Consultation codes were used to identify consultations when physicians were aware of the confirmatory nature of the consultation. The patient was seeking a second or third opinion. Physicians are now instructed to use the appropriate consultation code.

Online learning tools

CMS developed a learning tool that is available on disk. Some Medicare carriers may have the learning tool available online. It is a review of appropriate CPT coding. It takes approximately 20 minutes to navigate through the program. To receive the disk or determine whether your Medicare carrier offers the tool online, contact your local Medicare carrier.

CMS-sponsored E/M seminars

The medical review departments of your local Medicare carrier present these seminars. These sessions are a great avenue for asking questions directly of the medical review personnel who audit your documentation. Often, the carrier medical director attends these sessions as well. If your carrier is not currently offering the sessions, it may put one together specifically for your group. Contact your local Medicare carrier for more information.

Physician Regulatory Issues Team (PRIT)

CMS has put together this team to help clarify issues for physicians. For additional information and contacts, see the PRIT Web address on p. 204.

Helpful resources

- E/M documentation and guidelines
    - Go to *www.cms.hhs.gov/physicians* and scroll down to the section on coding. You will find a link there to the guidelines.
    - Levinson, Stephen R., MD. Practical E/M—*Documentation and Coding Solutions for Quality Patient Care*, American Medical Association Press, December 2005.
- Society of Hospital Medicine
    - *www.hospitalmedicine.org*
- Pay for performance
    - *www.cms.hhs.gov/apps/media/press/release.asp?Counter=1343*
- Recovery audit contractors
    - *http://new.cms.hhs.gov/MedlearnMattersArticles/downloads/SE0565.pdf*
- Critical care

- Society of Critical Care Medicine: *www.sccm.org/index.asp*

- Medline Plus—Critical Care: *www.nlm.nih.gov/medlineplus/criticalcare.html*

• **Progressive corrective action**

- *www.cms.hhs.gov/MedicalReviewProcess/02_progressivecorrectiveaction.asp*

• **Physician Regulatory Issues Team (PRIT)**

- *www.cms.hhs.gov/PRIT/PRITI/list.asp*

• **Medicare carrier contact numbers**

- To find toll fee numbers for contacting your Medicare carrier, go to *www.cms.hhs.gov/medlearn/tollnums.asp* and follow the directions provided at the bottom of the page.

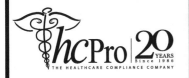

SAVE 20% ON RELATED HCPRO PRODUCTS!

Cash in your savings at **www.hcmarketplace.com**

Simply enter your source code MRELATED20 at checkout

Best-selling resources

Hospitalist Management Advisor

Need-to-know news, information, and best practices!

The monthly newsletter **Hospitalist Management Advisor** offers the latest and greatest in hospitalist management strategies and techniques.

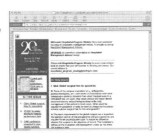

You'll learn directly from other successful hospitalist programs what works and what doesn't. You'll also receive tips and information on the topics that matter most to your professional success. Start your subscription today!

The Hospitalist Program Management Guide

Ensure your hospitalist program is a worthwhile investment!

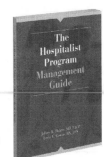

A surefire resource you'll consult often, **The Hospitalist Program Management Guide** will help your organization create, monitor, and assess the value of your hospitalist program. You'll learn how to measure your program's quality and effectiveness; ensure satisfaction of patients, primary care physicians, and hospital administration; secure hospitalists' loyalty; and more!

Hospitalist Program Weekly

Get the latest news, tips, tools, and regulatory updates delivered right to your inbox— absolutely FREE!

Access the very latest information, timely tips, techniques, and "tools of the trade" in our informative e-mail newsletter. *Hospitalist Program Weekly* will keep you on the cutting edge of critical hospitalist management issues.

Hospitalist Manual:
Evidence-based Approach to Medicine

Step-by-step training manual on evidence-based best practices for inpatient physicians.

Distributed by HCPro and produced by National Health Information LLC, the 350-page **Hospitalist Manual** will help busy physicians simplify their jobs and maximize their effectiveness in managing multiple clinical and managerial tasks.

The HCPro Risk-Free, Money-Back Guarantee
If for <u>any</u> reason you're not completely satisfied with your purchase, return it and you will receive a prompt, polite, 100% refund—*no questions asked*. **We guarantee it!**

(The following guarantee applies to specific product types: Books 30-day, videos 7-day, newsletters 100% guarantee)